LONG
DISTANCE
CAREGIVING

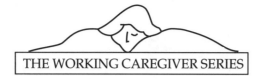

THE WORKING CAREGIVER SERIES

LONG DISTANCE CAREGIVING

*A Survival Guide
for Far Away Caregivers*

. . . .

Angela Heath, M.G.S.

ADVISORY PANEL
Evelyn Aker
Terry Freeman
Lynn Friss
Barbara Greenberg
Linda Jackson
Joan Kuriansky
Lorraine Lidoff
Robyn Stone

 AMERICAN SOURCE BOOKS

Lakewood • Colorado

Copyright © 1993 by Angela Heath

Series logo by Karen Groves
Cover design by Steven Phillips
Photographs by Ron Thornton

ATTENTION ORGANIZATIONS AND CORPORATIONS:
This book is available at quantity discounts on bulk purchases for educational, business, or sales promotional use. For further information, please contact American Source Books, PO Box 280353, Lakewood, CO 80228, (303) 980-0580.

Library of Congress Cataloging-in-Publication Data

Heath, Angela.
    Long distance caregiving : a survival guide for far away caregivers / Angela Heath.
        p. cm. -- (The Working caregiver series)
    Includes index.
    ISBN 0-9621333-9-6 : $9.95
    1. Aged--Care--United States. 2. Caregivers--United States. 3. Aged--United States--Family relationships. I. Title.
II. Series.
HV1461.H43 1991
362.6--dc20   92-42895

Printed and bound in the United States of America

Acknowledgements

. . . .

I would like to first and foremost thank God, my Father, for the inspiration and strength to complete this book.

To Steven Phillips, whose laid-back attitude, timely response and vision to pursue this title, a huge thanks. It has been a pleasure to work with you.

To my soul mate, Roger, thanks for your patience, encouragement and those constant reminders to work instead of play. Having you in my life made this project easier to complete.

Mom and Dad, what can I say. Thanks for your support through the years. I know you sometimes wonder about my decision making abilities. This book is for you.

To the caregivers who shared their stories — Ron, Kurt, Margaret, Barbara, Joyce, Mable, Jonas, Donna, Leslie Jean, Lincoln and Erica — thank you for the love you give to those in need. I hope I was able to help you cope.

I would also like to thank my review panel: Evelyn Aker, Terry Freeman, Lynn Friss, Barbara Greenberg, Joan Kuriansky, Lorraine Lidoff, Linda Jackson and Robyn Stone. Your suggestions helped to fine-tune the book.

FOREWORD

· · · · · · · · ·

As LIFE EXPECTANCY INCREASES, FERTILITY DECLINES, AND MORE
women enter the labor force; and as mobility increases both in
the developing and the developed countries for reasons of
upward mobility and survival, the traditional and the not so
traditional family are faced with the necessity to look after
aging family members from afar. Afar can mean across town,
across the country, or even across the ocean.

It has become rarer in today's world that family members
live in close proximity to one another. In our country sometimes
it is the older generation that moves away from their longtime
home—the city, town, or rural setting where they lived, raised
children, and worked until retirement. They might move to
Florida or some other sunbelt state. Or the children may move
to pursue jobs or careers, marry, or go away to college and
remain in the area of their schooling. Whatever the reason,
more families are scattered geographically. Not just families in
the industrialized countries, but even in the developing
countries where, for example, African villages have seen the
young people leave in droves to pursue work, education, even
just to survive, leaving behind the elderly.

Thus, there are many people who are trying to care for an
older family member from some distance away. Many are not
only far away, but many of the carers have time constraints
brought on by work, family, and children that must also be
accommodated. In work I have done previously with
caregivers, the most important thing they say they need is
information—and that is certainly doubly true for those who
are caring for someone far away—usually a place where they,
the carers, may not be familiar with what is available to aid them

in this endeavor. The second most important thing after information is organization...how to organize your efforts. This book is just what you need to help you (1) find the information you need in a distant city or state and (2) organize your efforts and assess your loved one's needs from afar.

I worked with Angela Heath on several caregiving projects when she worked at the American Association of Retired Persons (AARP). She has in-depth knowledge of the needs of caregivers, is sensitive to the needs of those being cared for, knows where to get information and how to direct you to it. In addition, she presents in this book the organizational framework to help you go about your tasks. As I know from personal experience, having taken care of both my mother and father, information and organization can mitigate panic and help you to feel more in charge of the situation which, no matter how simple or difficult, is bound to be fraught with emotion.

Elizabeth K. Mullen, Director
International Activities
American Association of Retired Persons
Washington, DC
November 1992

CONTENTS

Chapter One

SO, YOU'RE A CAREGIVER

. . . .

IF YOU ARE READING THIS BOOK, ODDS ARE YOU ARE LIKE millions of other Americans who are concerned about providing assistance to an aging spouse, parent, other relative, or friend. Your situation, in addition, is complicated by distance.

You are probably struggling with many difficult issues right now as you attempt to understand the older person's needs, make arrangements to meet those needs, and work with other family members and agencies that provide services. For a number of reasons, you may be feeling stressed, pressured, exhausted, and bewildered. You may be facing enormous telephone and travel bills in addition to other direct expenses related to providing care. You may be feeling intense conflicting emotions about the many different roles you must assume as caregiver; or possibly your relationship with the elder person and other caregivers may be strained. In all likelihood, you have other demands for your time and attention such as a spouse, children, job responsibilities, or your own health concerns.

If you can see yourself in any of these situations, then *Long Distance Caregiving: A Survival Guide for Far Away Caregivers* is your road map through the wilderness. This book will identify specific steps you can take to make long distance caregiving more manageable. Throughout the book, you are instructed to complete a number of basic tasks in preparing for a planned visit with the older person, or what is referred to as a "care commute" throughout the book. These tasks are designed to lay the groundwork for successful long distance caregiving.

A word of caution. This book is based on a planning model, and planning takes time, often more than originally thought. Prioritize the tasks you need to complete and address the most important tasks first. You will probably find that a few issues suggested in the book do not apply to your situation. These assignments should not add to your stress. Do not feel pressured into thinking that you must complete all of these tasks during one visit. You may need to make several visits or stay with the older person for an extended period of time in order to put supports in place.

There are a couple of things you will want to keep in mind in order to use this book most effectively. First, when possible, you will want to read this book in the order in which it is presented, as each chapter builds on the next. Avoid the temptation of starting with a chapter that seems most applicable to your current situation. If you are dealing with a crisis and you do not have time to read the entire book, you may want to read the introduction and summary to each chapter. Then, as you have more time available, you will know which chapters are most important for your situation.

Chapters 2 through 6 cover information you will want to become familiar with prior to your care commute. These chapters will help you identify and prioritize what you need to accomplish during your visit. Chapter 7 covers the actual visit and chapter 8 covers how to adjust your plan of care. In chapter 9, you will find helpful information on housing options for older persons. The final chapter discusses caring for someone who lives in another country.

Throughout the book, you are asked to record information in a Care Log. A Care Log is an easy-to-use, concise record of the important information you will need throughout your caregiving career. It contains all of the forms and exercises you will need to develop a plan of care for your older relative. American Source Books has Care Logs available for your convenience. You can purchase yours by calling (303) 980-0580 or by filling in and returning the order form at the back of this book.

Throughout the book, reference is made to the older person as a female. Hopefully, this does not distract you from valuable information if you are caring for a male. The female pronoun is used because receivers of care, just like caregivers, are overwhelmingly female. Likewise, the term "older relative" is used in many instances. Again, if you are the spouse, friend, or neighbor of the aging person who needs assistance, know that your contributions are recognized. It was just easier to describe the older person in these terms.

This book presumes that the reader is the one with primary responsibility for the older person. This may not always be the case. If you are not the primary caregiver, you may want to send a copy of this book to the person shouldering most of the responsibility. That way, you will both understand the tasks to be accomplished and how the work load should be divided.

In many instances, caregiving is a family affair. Yet family caregiving may not be all that easy. You, the older person, family members, other concerned persons, and paid care providers may all disagree about the course of action to take. Old difficulties and hurts may resurface and cause family decision making to be impossible. The older person may be obstinate and resist your help. These are just some of the trying family dynamics of caregiving.

Two important things to keep in mind. First, the older person should retain as much decision making ability as possible. Remember, your primary objective is to help the older person fulfill her needs, not to take over your relative's life. In some situations, when the older person is unable to make decisions, you may need to do so on her behalf. But if at all possible, allow the older person to control her destiny.

Second, family difficulties are typical. Very few families manage to come together in caregiving situations without some disagreement. Be honest about your family situation. Be realistic about what can be expected in terms of a familial approach to the older person's needs. Try different, non-threatening strategies to solicit cooperation among all concerned parties. If after trying different strategies you find that the family is still unable to function effectively, you may need the assistance of a professional.

A family therapist, social worker, or geriatric care manager can work with you and your family to solve issues and help the family function as a unit. These professionals can help you by conducting your family meeting, providing family and individual counseling, assessing the needs of the older person, and recommending services that would be useful. In addition, they can advise you concerning the financial resources available to pay for services.

One final note. It is important to remember that as a caregiver you need to understand the limits on what you can do personally. Allow others to help you. Traveling frequently to care for your relative can take its toll. Remember to take time out to care for yourself!

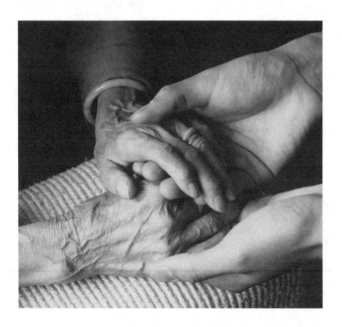

Chapter Two

SOME BASIC TECHNIQUES

· · · · · · · · ·

"I thought something was wrong with Mom: she didn't quite sound like herself—her voice sounded kind of weak. But, every time I asked her if things were OK she'd say yes. Then, one day while we were speaking on the telephone, she suddenly stopped talking. I kept saying, 'Mom, Mom, Mom, are you alright?' But she didn't answer. My wife and I immediately jumped in the car and drove three hours to her home. When we arrived, there she was, slumped over—she had blacked out. The doctor said she was suffering from malnutrition and dehydration."

—*Jonas, retired banker, age 62*

KNOWING IF AN OLDER PERSON IS HAVING A PROBLEM WHEN you live in a distant city or state can be difficult. At times, it may seem that the elder refuses to admit a problem and at other times, she may seem to exaggerate every small difficulty. And the way families respond to the needs of their distant relative varies a great deal too. Some caregivers are filled with anxiety, imagining the worst and over-reacting to insignificant conditions. Others are oblivious to major changes and concerns experienced by the older person.

Many times, caregivers and care receivers will differ in their perceptions. Is a concern a problem or not?. Is it a small or significant problem? These are the types of questions that cause long distance caregivers to lose a lot of sleep.

As a caregiver, you must understand that people experience changes and limitations as they grow older. Many of these changes may be a source of concern for you, but quite often the person experiencing the changes adjusts to them beautifully. It means that your older loved one may be willing to put up with minor inconveniences in order to maintain independence. It is your responsibility as a caring family member to allow the older person to find creative ways to adapt to these changes according to her own style. So, if things don't seem perfect, be sure they require your attention before you interfere.

This chapter helps by listing tips on how to get a feel for the older person's physical and emotional well-being over the telephone, keep the cost of long distance telephone bills to a minimum, communicate with the elder about sensitive issues, identify an informal network of support in the elder's community, and determine whether an in-person visit is needed.

HOW TO START

Start by purchasing a Care Log, a workbook that you will use to gather and organize information about your caregiving situation. You can either buy a Care Log with pre-printed worksheets (see order form at the back of the book), or you can build your own. If you decide to build your own, buy a spiral notebook or three-ring binder and divide it into the following sections:

Assessment—Under this section, keep notes about your relative's status. This would include your perceptions, those of others, and problems reported by the elder.

Medical Information—Gather data on the senior's medical condition. List the names, addresses, and telephone numbers for all medical and health personnel involved in the person's care. List all medications and the name, address, and telephone number of your relative's pharmacy. Also, list all adaptive devices used such as a wheelchair, cane or shower chair. Make general statements regarding the person's ability to walk, use the bathroom, feed herself, and bathe.

Travel—This will be a small section that contains useful facts for arranging travel. Include in this section the names and telephone numbers of car rental companies, bus lines, trains, and airlines. Note discount fares offered, and restrictions that apply. Be sure to place a date next to all fares listed as they are subject to change numerous times.

Informal Network—Use this section to identify the names, addresses, and telephone numbers for all persons in the older person's support network. Record any special data regarding their relationship with your relative and how they provide assistance.

Community Resources—This section will become very large as time goes on. Record the name, address, and telephone number for each health or social service agency to whom you speak. Keep notes that describe the services offered, the application process, waiting lists, and fees.

Legal, Financial, and Insurance—List the name, address and telephone number of your relative's attorney, banker, financial planner, and insurance broker. List all legal documents such as wills; living wills; social security cards; birth, marriage, and divorce certificates; and power of attorney. Itemize all bank account numbers, stocks, property titles, and appraisals of valuables. Likewise, record the insurance information for auto, homeowner's, medical, and disability policies. If possible, keep a copy of these documents.

Miscellaneous—Record additional data in this section.

TELEPHONE SAVINGS

You probably stay in contact with your older relative most often by telephone. You may find it necessary to call once a week, or every other week, to uncover information to help you decide when your presence is required. In some cases, caregivers call the older person every day. Telephone calls can be short yet allow you to get answers to your questions if you are organized before making the call and keep the conversation on track. This does not mean, however, that you subject your relative to a series of bold, negative, offensive questions. Use a pleasant conversational tone and tactfully discuss issues of concern.

Paying for long distance telephone calls can be quite expensive. However, if you are concerned, you will lower your telephone bill by practicing the following tips:

- Order a telephone directory for your relative's city so you can avoid calling information.
- Organize your thoughts before calling. List each topic you want to discuss under the Miscellaneous section in your Care Log and be sure to cover all issues during the conversation.
- Call during off-peak hours. Check with your long distance service to find out when it is least expensive to call.
- Check with your long distance carrier to explore volume discount plans like "MCI's Family and Friends" program and "AT&T's Reach Out America."
- Schedule conference calls when several family members need to talk simultaneously. This will eliminate the need to make several long distance calls to individual family members. Run these calls like a business meeting; after all, time is money.
- Consider ordering AT&T's residential 800 service by calling (800) 327-9700 so that your relative and informal network members can reach you without paying for the call. Current fees are a $10 sign-up charge, $5.50 per month service fee, and 26¢ per minute for each call.

DISCUSSING SENSITIVE ISSUES

When attempting to get a feel for your relative's well-being, do not give the impression that you are trying to take over the person's life. Instead, use a relaxed approach so that your relative does not feel that her independence is threatened. Do not change your usual style of communication or you might come across as insincere. Remember, your relative may be willing to make certain sacrifices and adjustments in order to remain independent. Think through your approach before making telephone calls. Ask yourself how she will react to certain questions. Do you have an open, honest communication history, or does she frequently hide the truth so that you won't worry? Is your relative's memory sharp enough to communicate accurate information?

One adult daughter, Jennifer, suspected that her mother was not eating properly because she noticed a sudden weight loss. Here is the conversation Jennifer had with her mother regarding her mom's eating habits.

Jennifer: "Mom, I tried to prepare some stuffing with the turkey last Sunday, but mine never tastes as good as yours. Mom, what did you have for dinner on Sunday?"
Mother: "Oh, I just fixed a little something. I wasn't very hungry."
Jennifer: "Do you still fix those large meals the way you used to?"
Mother: "No, not since your father died. I just don't feel like cooking much anymore."
Jennifer: "So, what did you cook on Sunday?"
Mother: "Well, well I really don't remember. What did I prepare?"
Jennifer: "What did you have for dinner tonight?"
Mother: "Oh, just a light snack. I wasn't very hungry."
Jennifer: "Did you go out for dinner or stay at home?"
Mother: "I stayed here. I didn't go out."
Jennifer: "What did you prepare for dinner?"
Mother: "I prepared what I felt like eating. Why do you need to know what I ate? What did you eat?"
Jennifer: "Mom, I love you and I realize that cooking probably isn't as enjoyable since Dad died. But eating a good, nutritious meal is important. Anyway, when is the last time you talked to Bob?"

During this conversation, Jennifer is very gentle in her approach, yet very persistent about getting the information she needs. By the end of the conversation she concludes that three scenarios are possible. First, her mother is eating well and forgetting what she ate. Or, her mother is not eating properly due to depression, loneliness, or forgetfulness. Or finally, her mother simply does not want to discuss the issue. It is important that Jennifer continues to discuss the topic of nutrition with her mother, but maybe at a later date because her mother is getting agitated.

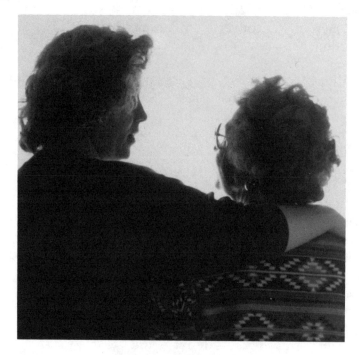

If Jennifer believes that the situation may be a serious safety or health concern that could result in a crisis, she may want to plan an immediate trip. However, if she feels that the situation is not serious, she should consult her mother's physician and gather additional details about her mom's health. It is important to note that some physicians will be more helpful than others. In some cases, you may find that your relative's doctor knows them quite well and is able to provide useful insights. In other cases, the doctor may not be able to tell you very much because your relative is being treated by several other physicians. Still in other cases, you will find that the physician is not good at talking with consumers. In addition, it may be necessary to have your relative sign a release of information form before you can get any information from the physician.

Here are some questions Jennifer may want to address:
- How much weight has her mother recently lost?
- What are past health conditions?
- Is her mom able to perform activities of daily living unassisted, i.e., eating, bathing, dressing, using the bathroom, and moving around in the house?
- Is she taking medications as directed?
- Are medications causing side affects?
- What happened at her last doctor's appointment?
- When was the last time her mother had her hearing and vision checked?
- Is she able to use adaptive equipment properly?
- How is she adjusting to recent life changes, i.e., retirement, death of a spouse, moving into a new home, or the inability to continue driving?
- Is she forgetting recent events or conversations?

When exploring the physical well-being of your older relative, you will want to enter your observations under the Assessment section of your Care Log. Be sure to give the doctor your telephone number and address.

IDENTIFYING AN INFORMAL NETWORK
In most cases, your relative has helpers and potential helpers in the community. Family and friends may help your relative from time to time, visit, run errands, and offer friendship. These people are your informal support network. As a caregiver, it is important that you identify members of your informal network and get a clear understanding of how they are willing to assist your relative. By gathering this data, you will have a better picture of your relative's situation and know who to contact for information.

Telephone your relative to begin identifying your informal support network. This network includes the following people who care about your relative:

- Persons currently helping your relative
- Relatives within a ten-mile radius
- Lifelong friends of yours and your relative
- Members of your relative's social or recreational clubs
- Good neighbors
- Members of churches and synagogues
- Members of religious organizations and institutions
- Physicians

Get telephone numbers, and addresses, if possible. Send a form letter to each person on your support list. (Writing helps cut down on the amount of time you will need to spend on the telephone with individual persons.) Address the letter to "Dear Friend." Explain that you are related to the older person and that you are concerned about your relative and would appreciate their assistance. Remember, these people care about your relative and, in most cases, they are more than willing to help. Include your address and telephone number and explain that you will be calling soon.

Next, call each person on your informal network list and discuss the following:

- Find out how each person is already involved with your relative.
- Ask someone your relative knows and feels comfortable with to call her twice a week.
- Ask someone your relative is fond of to visit at least once a week and to discreetly check around the house and observe your relative's appearance and behavior.
- Ask others to share meals with your relative, or simply make sure she gets out of the house from time to time.
- If necessary, ask someone your relative trusts to assist with paying bills, or have the bills forwarded to you.

- Provide them with your address and telephone number and encourage them to call you collect whenever needed.
- Ask them to drop you a note every now and then to let you know how your relative is doing.
- Let them know you will contact them in the near future.
- Show your appreciation for their kindness.

Include all the information you collect in the Informal Network section of your Care Log.

While constructing the support network, it is imperative that you work closely with your older relative and other concerned family members. In most cases, caregiving is a family affair with all members sharing in the decision-making. Again, your goal is to be nonthreatening and to help your older relative feel comfortable about any plan of support that the family develops.

In some cases, your relative may not have an informal network. She may have outlived family and friends, or they may have moved away. In these cases, it will be necessary to work with community agencies to get your relative's needs met. Further information of services for the elderly is contained in chapter 5.

NOTIFY YOUR EMPLOYER

You will want to let your employer know that you are dealing with a long distance caregiving situation. You may be able to work something out with your employer to make it easier for you to respond to emergency situations. In addition, your company may offer benefits that would be useful such as support groups or flexible use of leave time.

. . . .

This chapter provided you with some basic information to get you started completing important tasks. Nonetheless, keep in mind that long distance caregiving equals traveling. The next chapter takes up this important topic and will provide you with some valuable travel tips.

TO DO IN THE NEXT TWO WEEKS

✓ Purchase a Care Log by calling (303) 980-0580 or by filling out and returning the order form found at the back of the book; or, purchase a three-ring binder or spiral notebook and begin to build your own.

✓ Contact at least three long distance carriers and compare prices for telephone calls to your relative's city. Compare rates for daytime and evening calls. Switch to the least expensive carrier.

✓ Begin your telephone assessment of your relative's well-being by discussing health issues.

✓ Begin constructing your local support network by identifying family and friends who might assist.

✓ Order a telephone book for your relative's city by calling your local telephone company.

✓ Purchase a supply of thank-you cards to send to members of your support network.

✓ Contact your relative's physician regarding her overall health status.

✓ Ask your relative to read you the labels on all prescriptions. Call the pharmacist and talk about possible drug interactions.

✓ Draft your introductory letter for your support network.

✓ Contact AT&T at (800) 233-1222 for a brochure on products for the disabled.

✓ Contact your local department on aging to find out how you can join a caregiver support group, or attend a caregiver educational program.

Chapter Three

TRAVEL TIPS

· · · · · · · · ·

"I try to visit my mother at least twice a year. Normally, I plan my visits far enough in advance to save on airfare. There have been a couple times over the past three years when I have had to drop everything to go to Mother's side because she was sick. Those trips were very expensive. When I think about it, there was one time when I really didn't have to go, but I didn't know that at the time."

—*Donna, nutritionist, age 59*

CARE COMMUTING IS AN INEVITABLE REQUIREMENT FOR LONG distance caregiving. Traveling can be physically and mentally exhausting and it can be very expensive. Advance planning will allow you to explore the advantages and disadvantages of different modes of travel. However, there may be times when you are unable to plan due to an emergency. But what constitutes an emergency?

This chapter will help you avoid making unnecessary expensive trips. It will help you decide when you can postpone a visit to reduce your travel expenses. It reviews issues to consider regarding different modes of transportation, and it provides tips on how to get to your destination inexpensively. By following the suggestions provided in this chapter you will access useful travel information.

WHEN SHOULD YOU GO?

From a distance, you may not always know when a visit to your relative is necessary. It is a real challenge to make an accurate assessment of your relative's condition. Telephone conversations may not provide the answer because your relative may not paint an accurate description of the situation. Perhaps your relative does not want you to worry; or, perhaps she overdramatizes the situation because she wants your attention.

DEALING WITH AN EMERGENCY

What is an emergency? Clearly there are circumstances that obviously indicate an emergency. If you are confronted with any of the following scenarios, you will want to visit your relative immediately:

- A health professional requests your presence due to a serious medical condition.
- A calamity occurs, such as a fire or natural disaster.
- Family or friends report a sharp decline in the older person's physical health or mental status.
- No one has been able to contact the older person.
- Persons assisting your relative tell you that the older person has a number of unmet needs that detract from her health or safety.
- An accident occurs, such as a drug overdose, a car accident, or a fall that results in severe injury.

If you are faced with a crisis, you have two things in mind—get to your relative quickly and find a way to deal with the issues presented by the emergency. Be sure to take this book and your Care Log with you on your trip. You may not have time to read the next few chapters of this book; therefore, following are a few topics covered in the book that you may want to skim as time permits. The page numbers for each topic are provided so that you can go directly to the information you need. You may find that these topics can help you better respond to the emergency.

- Check with transportation providers regarding inexpensive rates (pages 29-32).
- Spend time coordinating the care your relative needs (pages 73-76).
- Learn about available services (pages 39-45).
- Investigate relocation options (pages 90-96).

These topics are just a few that might help you cope with a crisis. You will want to skim other sections of the book that address your needs. You are encouraged to read the entire book after the emergency has subsided.

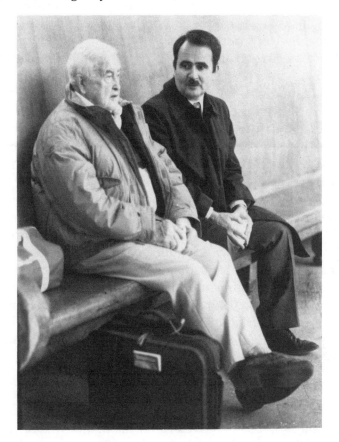

NONEMERGENCY SITUATIONS

When you are not dealing with a crisis, for the most part you must rely on the older person's perception of the problem, and the perception of others with whom she has contact. Generally, you have a good idea of whether your older relative has a tendency to exaggerate, cover up, or manipulate you so you will come for a visit. Also, you know your own tolerance level. Some care providers would be guilt-ridden if they suspected their relative was experiencing some difficulty and they delayed rushing to the rescue. Others can logically deduce that the situation does not demand immediate attention and are able to live with that line of reasoning. Be aware that this approach could backfire if you decide to delay a trip and the situation develops into a crisis.

Here are two examples of how caregivers applied these different approaches:

Lisa found out that her mother had been diagnosed with cancer earlier in the day. Although her mother was feeling fine and her father was there to console her, Lisa immediately notified her supervisor that she had a family emergency and headed for her mother's house, five hours away. You may be thinking that this situation did not demand immediate attention as Lisa's father was there and Lisa could speak with her mother over the telephone every day until she could plan a trip in the next few weeks. For Lisa, nonetheless, it was important to be there and to provide emotional support.

Jessica's mother was diagnosed with lung cancer. Her mother was also feeling fine but did not have a spouse available to provide emotional support. Jessica immediately began calling family and friends and arranged for them to visit her mother. She talked with her mother's physician and began collecting information on her mother's condition and prognosis. She then wrote down what she thought needed to be discussed with her mother and began to think about possible future needs based on her mother's prognosis. Jessica drove to her mother's house two weeks after the diagnosis. For Jessica, it was more important to do as much background work as possible so that when she made her visit, she was more prepared to launch a plan of action. She felt that her mother had enough emotional support and that a phone call every night before her visit was sufficient.

In a nonemergency situation, you will need to consider a number of issues when deciding whether a trip can be delayed. Following are some areas that might influence your decision to travel now or later.

- Can someone else complete the caregiving tasks? Can you rely on your informal network to take care of the situation?
- Can you financially afford the trip? How much money would you save on travelling expenses by delaying your trip for a couple of weeks? Can you afford to travel and still meet your financial obligations at home?
- Do you have leave time available at work? If not, can you afford to take leave without pay? Do you need to make arrangements to have work completed in your absence?
- Do you need to make special arrangements for your children and/or spouse?
- Do you need to complete certain business transactions before your trip, such as transferring money and paying bills?
- Do you anticipate needing to visit your relative again in the near future? If so, can you comfortably make two trips within a short time period?
- What would be the consequences of not visiting your relative?

Once you have decided whether the situation demands your immediate attention, or how long you can delay a personal visit, decide how you want to travel.

HOW TO GET THERE

Begin to figure out the best way to get there. Travelling by car may be ideal for a short trip of four hours or less. Trains and buses are alternatives if they provide quick service to your relative's city at reasonable prices. Air travel may be the only choice when you need to get there quickly and your relative lives hundreds of miles away. In investigating the best mode of transportation for your situation, call for information at night when reservationists are not so busy.

If you prefer to travel by car, consider the following issues:

- Have your car inspected by a reputable mechanic to make sure it is in good condition for the trip.
- Contact a motorist club like AAA to check on the road and weather conditions.
- If you do not have a car available, ask to rent a friend's car for less than car rental companies charge per day and without a mileage charge. Make sure your friend has full insurance coverage and agree, in advance, on how you would handle theft or accidents.
- If renting a car is your only option, let automobile rental companies know that you are dealing with a family crisis or that you are a hardship case. You may be able to secure a discounted rate.
- Compare the different rates offered by rental car companies. Ask for your company's corporate rate and find out about discount rates for organizations and auto/travel clubs to which you may belong.
- Figure out how many miles you plan to travel. Either find a company that provides a high number of free miles or one that does not charge daily mileage.
- If you have full insurance coverage on your personal car, waive all insurance offered by auto rental companies. Your insurance will cover you.
- Be sure to fill the gas tank of your rental car before returning it.
- When possible, plan trips to take advantage of weekend car rental discounts from Thursday to Monday.
- Avoid driving if you are too upset or tired.

If you prefer to travel by bus or train, consider the following issues:

- Call several bus and train companies to investigate the average price of tickets to your relative's city, how long it takes to get there, and how many stops you will make. Ask them to send you a schedule.
- Let the bus or train company know that you are dealing with a family crisis or that you are a hardship case. You may be able to secure a discounted rate.
- Check for special rates, like Amtrack's All Aboard America Fare, and check to see if the rates vary according to the hour of departure.
- Compare the price of fare passes, like Greyhound's Ameri-Pass, which allows you to travel anytime for a certain number of days, with regular or discounted fares.

If you prefer to travel by airplane, consider the following issues:

- Let the airline know that you are dealing with a family crisis or that you are a hardship case. Although there were no bereavement rates during the time this book was written, airfares and airline policies can change quickly.
- If possible, try to purchase your ticket at least seven days in advance to get a decreased rate.
- Plan your trip so that you can stay over a Saturday night, thereby getting a fare break.
- Purchase coupons for seniors, if you are eligible, and use them to travel standby during an emergency situation.
- Join an airline frequent flyer club. Use one carrier as often as possible to earn miles toward a free or discounted ticket.
- Look for inexpensive tickets in the classified section of the newspaper.

BEFORE YOU LEAVE

Before you begin your care commute, read chapters 4 through 7. These chapters contain specific information to help you plan the tasks you hope to complete. Study the chapters that will help you with your primary concerns and complete the suggested activities. After reading these chapters, you will understand your role, the resources to assist you, and the approach to use.

Remember, you need not attempt to complete all of these tasks alone. Get members of your informal support network to help you. Go to your Care Log and review your notes. Identify the top concerns that you want to focus on during your visit. Ask members of your support network to verify your perceptions and to help you identify community organizations that can provide assistance. Discuss with them possible options for addressing these problems. Schedule appointments with several members of your network early during your trip to solicit additional information and to develop close working relationships. If possible, treat these persons to breakfast, lunch, or simply a cup of coffee.

Select one issue to address for every two days you plan to visit. You will find that it takes time to adequately deal with caregiving problems and to put a responsive care plan in place. Realize that additional concerns will surface while you are visiting. Simply add new concerns to your list and select the top issues to address during this trip. If possible, avoid attempting to address all problem areas during your stay. Consider saving less important issues for a later trip. This will help you stay focused and avoid frustration.

. . . .

In this chapter you explored when it is necessary to visit your relative and the best way to get there. In the next chapter, you will learn about services that may be available in your relative's community.

TO DO TWO WEEKS BEFORE TO YOUR TRIP

In some cases, particularly medical emergencies, you will not have the luxury of time to prepare for your trip. Nonetheless, when you have the time to schedule a trip, you will want to accomplish the following goals before you travel.

✓ Read chapters 4 through 7 before your care commute.

✓ Decide how long you can delay a personal visit in order to do some advance planning.

✓ Explore various transportation options and decide which option is most feasible.

✓ Notify your support network of your travel plans and schedule meetings with key players.

✓ Notify your older relative of your travel plans and ask her to begin gathering the documents you will need. Ask her to put them together in a safe place.

✓ Select your primary issues of concern and begin identifying people you want to contact during your care commute.

✓ Write thank-you cards for members of your support network who were especially helpful.

✓ Start a caregiver emergency fund to pay for your travel expenses and other expenses you might incur.

Chapter Four

THE AGING NETWORK

· · · · · · · · ·

"I had never heard of an 'aging network.' I knew about the meals program that comes to older people's homes because my wife heard about it from one of her friends. I didn't even know where to call first. Luckily, my wife called one of her friends who was dealing with her sick mother and she told my wife to contact this organization for senior citizens. My wife called them and they told her to call somewhere else. After about three or four long distance calls, she was in the 'aging network' and we were able to get some assistance with my mother."

—Lincoln, retired military, age 65

THE AGING NETWORK HAS JOKINGLY BEEN REFERRED TO AS "the invisible network" by caregivers who are frustrated with trying to gain access to services. Like Lincoln, many long distance caregivers do not know where to start because they are unaware of the numerous programs and services available in their relative's community. Many caregivers agree that once you are in the system it is much easier to identify agencies and individuals to help; but gaining access to the system can be time-consuming, frustrating and confusing.

The aging network is a national system of organizations that provide services to elderly persons and their families. It includes federal, state, regional, and local agencies. Unfortunately, the services available throughout this system vary from location to location. Consequently, long distance caregivers can easily get confused because programs that they heard about in their own community may not be available in the community where their older relative lives.

In this chapter, you will learn all about the aging network—what it is, how to access it, and the services available to help you. You will also learn the proper names for services so that you can communicate effectively with service providers.

THE AGING NETWORK

The aging network consists of a federal office; state departments; over 670 regional aging offices; and thousands of county, city, and local agencies that provide services to the elderly and their families. The network was established by the federal Older Americans Act of 1965. The Act was created to ensure that older Americans enjoy the following benefits:

- Adequate retirement income
- The best physical and mental health
- Suitable housing
- Restorative services for those requiring institutional care
- Opportunity for employment
- Meaningful civic, cultural, and recreational opportunities
- Available community services that provide assistance in a coordinated manner
- Immediate benefit from research
- Freedom in planning and managing their own lives

The Older Americans Act is administered by the Administration on Aging (AoA), a federal agency located in Washington, DC. AoA is responsible for a number of duties including serving as a clearinghouse for information related to aging, administering funds provided by the Act, disseminating educational materials, and training professionals. But most important to caregivers is the responsibility of providing technical assistance and grants to state and local agencies to develop comprehensive and coordinated service systems for older persons.

State Units on Aging (SUAs) receive funding from AoA to develop a state plan that coordinates all state activities related to the Act. There is a State Unit on Aging in every state and each U.S. territory. In most cases, states funnel federal dollars to smaller planning and service areas called Area Agencies on Aging (AAA). (In several states, the SUA is also the AAA.) AAAs undertake the planning and provision of services in their designated areas. These agencies are required by law to offer information and referral services, i.e., provide information to citizens and refer them to appropriate service providers. AAAs contract with numerous local agencies that provide services for the elderly.

You will want to start with the AAA in your older relative's area, or the local city or county department on aging. Refer to the government section in the telephone book for your relative's community under "aging" or "senior citizens." Or, you can use a new service offered by the National Association of Area Agencies on Aging called the Eldercare Locator. This service will provide you with the telephone number and mailing address of the AAA that covers your relative's area and, in some cases, the community resource that can best meet your needs. You can reach the Eldercare Locator Service by calling (800) 677-1116. Be sure to have your relative's address available for the Eldercare Locator operator.

ACCESSING THE SERVICE SYSTEM

Once you have located the aging network, you will still need to gain access to the services you need. This can be a confusing and frustrating ordeal. Have your Care Log ready and take copious notes as you use the following tips to guide you through the maze of aging services:

- Start by making investigative telephone calls.
- Call early in the morning if you need a quick response. By calling during lunchtime, it is quite possible that the person you need to speak with will be out and will therefore have to return your call and pay for the charges.

- Mentally prepare yourself to deal with the possibility of being transferred, disconnected, or referred to other persons several times before you reach the person who can help you.
- Use an upbeat, friendly, yet assertive tone.
- Introduce yourself and get the name and direct telephone number of everyone you contact.

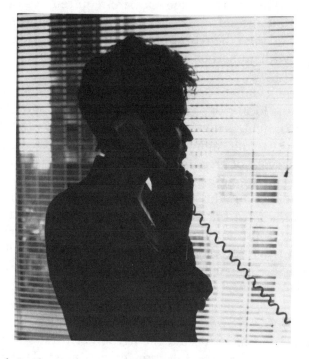

- Explain that you are a long distance caregiver. If you are calling long distance, be sure to let them know.
- Ask to speak with a case manager or social worker if possible. These persons can help you sort through issues to uncover hidden or unidentified needs your relative may have.
- Explain your needs as clearly as possible.
- Ask questions about eligibility criteria, waiting lists, fees for services, and various options for meeting your needs.

- Ask that program information and applications be mailed or faxed to you and/or your relative.
- If necessary, schedule a face-to-face interview. Make a list of documents you need to bring with you. Get directions to the agency if needed.
- Before hanging up, repeat the information you have received to verify your understanding of the issues discussed.
- Ask if there are other organizations you should contact, or if the worker has any other helpful suggestions.
- Be courteous and extend a hearty "thank you" to persons who have been helpful. Flattery just might get you where you want to go.
- Report discourteous, rude workers to their supervisors.

Once you have completed your investigative telephone calls, you will want to complete the follow-up instructions you received. You should have several pages of organizations to contact about specific services. The following sections provide an overview of the kinds of services that may be available in your relative's community. Services can be broken down into those that are offered in the community and those that are delivered to the home.

SERVICES DELIVERED IN THE COMMUNITY
The following services, offered in the community, may be useful for long distance caregivers. Sometimes, senior transportation services will take elders to the site and escorts will assist with boarding the bus or van. Again, you may find that some of these services are not available in your relative's community.

Nutrition Sites
Nutrition sites offer noontime meals in a central location such as a senior center, church or synagogue, community center, or housing project. Caregivers know that elders are receiving a nutritious meal and socializing with peers when they attend nutrition sites.

Senior Centers

At these centers, seniors can participate in recreational, health, and educational programs. Often centers are able to connect seniors and caregivers with other services available in the community.

Adult Day Care

An adult day care center is a place that provides a supportive and therapeutic environment for seniors with mental or physical limitations. A range of health, social, nutritional and educational programs is provided. Centers typically operate between normal business hours and are offered by hospitals, religious organizations, and other nonprofit groups.

Congregate Living Facilities

This type of senior housing offers independent living, central dining, and a host of recreational and health programs. Seniors who are able to live independently but want the security of knowing that support is available when needed are ideal candidates for this type of housing. Rents vary greatly from location to location. Facilities subsidized by the federal government for moderate-income seniors and handicapped persons require residents to pay no more than one-third of their income for rent.

Assisted Living Facilities

Sometimes referred to as board and care homes, these houses provide a room, meals, medication supervision, assistance with personal care, and 24-hour supervision. These facilities are ideal for seniors who are unable to care for themselves without supervision and assistance.

IN HOME SERVICES

The following services, offered in the home, may be useful to long distance caregivers:

Personal Emergency Response Systems (PERS)

These systems allow an older person to transmit a signal of distress to emergency telephone numbers. PERS can be devices worn around the neck or devices placed in the bathroom or bedroom. Either way, PERS provide seniors and caregivers with an added sense of security.

Homemakers

Homemaker aides assist with light housework, laundry, ironing, and cooking. Homemaker services are offered by private agencies, nonprofit organizations, religious groups, and family service organizations. Fees vary and may be offered on a sliding scale basis, i.e., based on the senior's ability to pay.

Home Health Care

Home health care includes a variety of health services that are brought into the home. Medical services provided by professional nurses or therapists, and personal care services, like bathing and grooming, provided by home health aides are two examples of home health care. Services are offered by private agencies and nonprofit organizations.

Chore Services

Chore services are frequently offered by religious organizations and nonprofit groups. They provide assistance with heavy housework such as mowing the lawn, shoveling snow,and washing windows.

Telephone Reassurance

A person, usually a volunteer, calls an elder every day at a predetermined time. If the elder does not answer the call, emergency contacts are telephoned.

Friendly Visitors

Sometimes referred to as senior companions, visitors provide socialization. They can write letters, read books, play games, or simply talk with the senior.

Home-Delivered Meals

Often referred to as "Meals-on-Wheels," these programs deliver hot noontime meals and sometimes a cold snack to a senior's home during the weekdays. A few programs offer weekend service. Costs vary and some programs accept donations in any amount.

Care Management

This service helps caregivers determine the needs of older persons with multiple problems and locate appropriate services. Care management services are offered by local departments on aging, hospitals, and private practitioners.

Care management services are very useful for caregivers who are unable to develop a plan of care for their relative. The local department on aging in your relative's area will be able to connect you with publicly-funded care management services. Private geriatric care managers charge fees for their services. You can locate a private care manager by contacting the National Association of Private Geriatric Care Managers at 655 N. Alvernon Way, Suite 108, Tucson, AZ 86711, (602) 881-8088.

ADDITIONAL SERVICES

There are other organizations that provide services for older persons and their family members. Disease-specific organizations such as the Alzheimer's Association and the Arthritis Foundation have helpful information and sponsor useful programs. Also, check with organizations like the local United Way, churches and synagogues, community service agencies, and family service agencies to locate additional services.

PAYING FOR SERVICES

All of the services under the Older Americans Act are available to Americans 60 years of age or older without charge, or for a modest fee. There often is a fee for other community services. In some cases, service agencies base their fees on a sliding scale basis, or according to the senior's ability to pay. In some limited cases, Medicare will cover adult day care, home health care, and medical transportation. Medicaid will pay for some community services if the older person meets specific financial guidelines. And, private health and long-term care insurance will pay for some services. You should talk with a social worker at the social service agency about your options for paying for services received.

KEEP ORGANIZED, AND PERSEVERE

Keep notes on the services available in your relative's community in the Community Resources section of your Care Log. You may not need to use some of these programs now but you may need them in the future. Create a "Resources in Place" page in the Community Resources section where you list information about the services your relative will start receiving. Include the

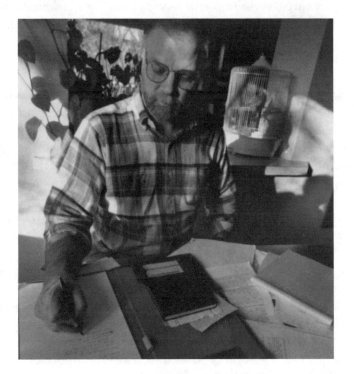

address and telephone number of a contact person at the agency providing each service. Make special notes about how the services will be delivered, how often, and by whom.

It is important to note that many of the services listed above may not be available in your relative's community. There are few services in many communities throughout the country, particularly in rural areas. Similarly, there are long waiting lists for services in many urban areas. If you have a need for a service and it is not available in your relative's community, you may be able to take an active role in advocating for the service. Talk with local service providers and politicians to get support for the service you feel is needed. Agree to testify at hearings, write letters, get others involved. With perseverance, you may be able to help establish a needed service.

Many caregivers choose to rely on family and friends when services are not available. Here is an example of how Margaret compensated for the lack of formal services in her father's community:

Margaret's father lives in a very small rural town where there are few social services. After she tried unsuccessfully to find a Meals-on-Wheels program, she finally asked the local restaurant owner if he would prepare meals for her father. He agreed and Margaret arranged for someone to pick up the meals. When it was obvious that her father could no longer live alone, she asked family friends to move in with her father. Later, Margaret did manage to find a paid personal care aide to assist with bathing and grooming. In addition, the man who cut her father's lawn was recruited to help with heavy lifting. This arrangement proved beneficial when Margaret's father fell and this man was able to lift him from the floor. Another family friend served as Margaret's key contact person. This person coordinated the other caregivers and provided regular reports to Margaret after she returned home.

Margaret's situation typifies the creativity caregivers must employ in developing a plan of care, particularly when services are not available.

MONITORING THE FORMAL SYSTEM

Once you have succeeded in getting a particular service started for your older relative, your worries are not over. From time to time there will be problems with the delivery of the service. In some cases, you will experience frequent problems. For example, home health aides may not show up or may not complete the tasks required. Likewise, senior transportation services may be an hour or two late picking up your relative for a doctor's appointment. In any case, both you and your relative will need to be assertive.

Talk with your older relative and make sure that she understands the services she can expect to receive, and how and when they should be delivered. Decide how you will respond to concerns about service delivery. Be sure to give your relative a copy of the "Resources in Place" page you created in case she needs to contact providers. Ask your relative to handle concerns directly. However, if they become too bothersome, you may need to handle the concerns yourself.

As mentioned in earlier chapters, make sure that every person or organization that has agreed to assist your relative has your name and telephone number, and vice versa. As mentioned in chapter 2, you will want to send them a letter to reiterate your understanding of how they have agreed to help. Thank them for their assistance and encourage them to call you collect occasionally to let you know how things are going.

. . . .

This chapter provided you with information on the aging network so that you can solicit appropriate services and thereby develop a care plan for your older relative. The next chapter will help you complete important paperwork.

TO DO IN THE NEXT TWO WEEKS

✓ Contact your local department on aging and speak with someone about your situation. Ask for insight and tips as to how you should approach the service system in your relative's community, and the types of services that may best fit your relative's needs.

✓ Call the Eldercare Locator Service at (800) 667-1116 to identify the local area agency on aging that covers your relative's area.

✓ Contact the area agency on aging in your relative's area to order a directory of services.

✓ Contact local service agencies and begin scheduling appointments.

✓ Order your free copy of *Making Wise Decisions for Long Term Care* (order #D12435) from AARP to learn more about services for the elderly. Write AARP, 601 E Street, NW, Washington, DC 20049.

✓ Order a free copy of *How to Choose a Home Care Agency* from the National Association for Home Care, 519 C Street N. E., Stanton Park, Washington DC 20002. Send a stamped, self-addressed legal size envelope with your request.

✓ Ask your employer about company benefits that would be helpful.

✓ Talk with your company's Employee Assistance Program staff if you are really worried about your relative.

Chapter Five

NECESSARY PAPERWORK

· · · · · · · · ·

"And the paperwork was a nightmare. Mom didn't know where anything was. She had never paid much attention to the bills, insurance or anything like that. In fact, she had never written a check. Can you imagine! So we had to start from scratch. Dad didn't really have any system to where he kept things. We must have looked through boxes and boxes of old papers to find what we needed... Dad, with Alzheimer's disease, was no help."

—*Mable, claims representative, age 58*

PAPERWORK IS ANOTHER INEVITABLE ELEMENT OF CAREGIVING. Service providers require financial information and completed forms. Health professionals require insurance information and completed medical forms. In addition, background information will be repeated on numerous forms. Consequently, you will want to locate all legal, financial, and insurance documents. As a caregiver, you will find these papers are required for many of the tasks you need to accomplish.

For long distance caregivers, this paperwork may be even more cumbersome. In most cases, locating, reviewing, and organizing documents is time-consuming and tedious. You may not know where certain information is located. You may feel pressured about dealing with so many papers and forms during a short stay. However, you will find that being organized will lessen some of the anxiety.

In this chapter, you will learn how to develop a step-by-step approach for identifying and locating important papers, how to organize these documents, and suggestions for storing important papers.

WHERE TO START

Hopefully, you are able to solicit the assistance of your older relative in locating and organizing documents. If you followed the advice given in chapter 3, you asked your relative to start locating records before your care commute. If she was able to do so, you are ahead of the game. In some cases, the older person will resist sharing personal information with the caregiver. You may need to convince this person that your only interest in examining these documents is to make it easier for you to provide and coordinate the assistance she needs now and in the future. If the person is still resistant, you may have to play a minimal role in organizing paperwork, like locating the documents and then making sure your relative knows how to update them.

While some older persons are very good at keeping and organizing important papers, others seem unable to locate needed documents. If this is the case, you may find yourself sorting through piles of papers located in many different places, both inside and outside of the house. Here are some places to look for important records:

✓ Scrapbooks
✓ File cabinets
✓ Dresser drawers, desk drawers, and closets
✓ Attic, garage, and basement
✓ Under the bed
✓ Safe deposit box
✓ Attorney's or accountant's office
✓ Another relative's home
✓ The home of the executor of the will

To help you organize your search, there are three useful work sheets in the Legal, Financial and Insurance section of your Care Log. The first work sheet itemizes the legal documents you need to locate, the second work sheet will be used to catalog financial documents, and the final work sheet itemizes insurance policies. Once you have attempted to locate these papers, you will want to write down the results of your search and any other important findings.

If you are creating your own Care Log, copy the following pages. Be sure to add entries for important papers your relative may possess that have not been noted in these examples.

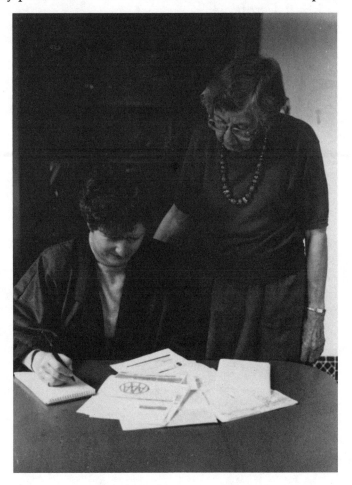

LEGAL DOCUMENTS

Status codes:

LA	*located and available*	C	*make a duplicate*
LN	*located but not available*	L	*lost, request duplicate*
UD	*needs to be updated*	N/A	*not applicable*
GD	*get document*		

Status	**Document**	**Comments**
	Birth Certificate	
	Social Security Card	
	Marriage License(s)	
	Divorce Decree(s)	
	Military Records	
	Will	
	Living Will	
	Power of Attorney	
	Health Care Power of Attorney	
	Legal Agreements	
	Other_____	
	Other_____	
	Other_____	

FINANCIAL DOCUMENTS

Status codes:

LA	located and available	C	make a duplicate
LN	located but not available	L	lost, request duplicate
UD	needs to be updated	N/A	not applicable
GD	get document		

Status	**Document**	**Account #**	**Company**
	Checking Account		

Contact (name, address, telephone):

Savings Account

Contact:

Retirement Account

Contact:

Stock Certificates

Contact:

Savings Bonds

Contact:

Real Estate Deed/Title

Contact:

Automobile Title

Contact:

Investment Income

Contact:

Other Income

Contact:

Other Income

Contact:

Other Income

Contact:

Mortgage Statement

Contact:

FINANCIAL DOCUMENTS *(Continued)*

Status	Document	Account #	Company
	Property Tax Statement		
Contact:			
	Lease Agreement		
Contact:			
	Hospital Bill		
Contact:			
	Doctor Bills		
Contact:			
	Utility Statement		
Contact:			
	Utility Statement		
Contact:			
	Telephone Bill		
Contact:			
	Credit Card		
Contact:			
	Credit Card		
Contact:			
	Credit Card		
Contact:			
	Other Debts		
Contact:			
	Other Debts		
Contact:			
	Other Debts		
Contact:			

INSURANCE DOCUMENTS

Status codes:

LA	*located and available*	*C*	*make a duplicate*
LN	*located but not available*	*L*	*lost, request duplicate*
UD	*needs to be updated*	*N/A*	*not applicable*
GD	*get document*		

Status	**Document**	**Policy #**	**Company**
	Auto		

Contact (name, address, telephone):

	Homeowner/Renters		

Contact:

Life Insurance

Contact:

Medicare

Contact:

Medicaid

Contact:

Medigap

Contact:

Long-term Care

Contact:

Disability

Contact:

Liability

Contact:

Other

Contact:

Other

Contact:

Other

Contact:

You will notice that there is a set of codes at the beginning of each page. These codes should be used in the status column to designate what, if anything, needs to be done with each document. If appropriate, feel free to use as many codes as necessary for each document. Following are the complete explanations for the codes:

LA—You have located the record and it is currently available for your review.

LN—You know where the document is located but it is not currently available for your review. Make a notation about where the document is located.

UD—The document needs to be updated.

GD—You need to get one of these documents.

C—You need to make a duplicate. You will need at least one copy of each document to take home with you.

L—The record has been lost; you need to request a duplicate.

N/A—Not applicable. Your relative does not have or need this record.

After you have completed the Legal, Financial, and Insurance section of your Care Log, you will have a good idea of the documents at hand, those that are stored somewhere else, and the documents that need to be created. At this point, you will want to do three things: get the papers you need but do not currently have, update records, and file and store your papers.

LOCATING MISSING RECORDS

Locating missing documents may take a great deal of time. Start with the places and/or people you think have access to these papers. If the documents are not available through these sources, then contact the offices that issued the records. Record the addresses and telephone numbers of these offices. You can then telephone to find out what you have to do to get a duplicate record. Or, you can develop a form letter requesting that a copy be sent to your relative. Have your older relative sign the form letters and get them in the mail before you leave town.

You may not have time to locate each document that you need. Therefore, as always, prioritize. Which documents do you need now and which ones can wait until later? Also, can you ask a trusted member of your informal network to help you? This person can follow up with local offices to get duplicate records after you have returned home.

UPDATING RECORDS

Oftentimes, you will find that older persons have not updated important papers to reflect the changes that have occurred over the years. You and your relative will want to ask yourselves the questions listed below while the two of you examine the records you have gathered. Make a list in your Care Log of how these records need to be changed.

- Are the correct address and last name used on all documents?
- Is the will current in terms of the executor, beneficiaries, and distribution of assets?
- In case of emergency, should you or someone else be given access to bank accounts and other assets?
- Are all household bills paid up to date?
- Should a financial expert review the current investments?
- Are the correct beneficiaries listed on insurance policies?
- Are the amounts of various insurance benefits adequate?

If you find that certain records need to be updated, contact the institutions responsible for issuing the records. Follow their guidelines to make necessary changes.

SETTING UP A FILING SYSTEM

Once you have gathered these documents, they need to be stored in a safe place. But first, make copies of all documents to take with you when you leave. This will be a safeguard in case some information gets lost. You should avoid taking original documents home with you because your older relative will not have access to them when needed. You may want to categorize the papers the way they are listed: legal documents, financial papers and insurance policies. If possible, you will want to keep all of these records in the same place.

You and your relative will need to decide where the documents should be archived. The safest place to keep important documents is a safe deposit box. If you choose this option, be sure to note the bank where the records are being kept. Ask your relative if your name can be added to the signature card in case you need to access the safe deposit box during an emergency.

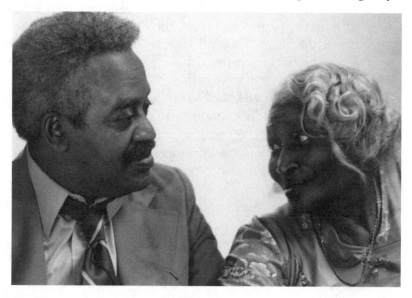

Your relative may prefer to keep the records at home for easy access. If so, make sure that important papers are kept in a fireproof box and that you know exactly where the documents are kept. You may also want to ask for the duplicate key to the box in case of emergency.

. . . .

In this chapter, you were shown a step-by-step approach for locating, updating, filing, and storing important documents you will need now or in the future. In the next chapter, you will review important legal, financial, and insurance issues.

TO DO IN THE NEXT TWO WEEKS

✓ Check with your relative to see how she is doing locating needed documents.

✓ Begin talking to your relative about which documents have and have not been located.

✓ Copy the legal, financial, and insurance pages from this chapter into your Care Log.

✓ Use the telephone book from your relative's area to identify print shops that are close to your relative's home and offer duplicating services.

✓ Contact Kelly Assisted Living at (800) 541-9818 for a free copy of "Organizing Records and Legal Considerations."

Chapter Six

LEGAL AND FINANCIAL ISSUES

. . . .

"Dealing with attorneys was a nightmare and a tremendous expense even though the lawyer we used was a family friend. Mother was not very cooperative at first, she thought we were conspiring against her. She's starting to get kind of forgetful. There were times when I didn't know what was going on—Mother was just signing papers and I was just signing papers...I wish we would have talked with an attorney before Mother started to get sick."

—Erica, homemaker, age 61

FOR MOST CAREGIVERS, LEGAL AND FINANCIAL ISSUES ARE IN-timidating topics. Few people know much about the legal instruments and financial options available to them and their older relative. And, as most caregivers come face to face with these issues during a crisis, decisions must be made quickly, which often allows little time to review options.

Preplanning helps decrease much of the frustration associated with legal paperwork and financial management and helps you avoid making costly errors. This chapter will review legal instruments that can make your job easier. It will discuss financial choices and explain options to pay for long-term care.

THE VALUE OF ADVANCE PLANNING

Financial and legal planning are difficult subjects to discuss. For some, to do so is an indication that something bad is about to happen. Others hesitate because many of the issues that need to be considered and discussed are quite sensitive. Some seniors resist preplanning because they do not want to share their financial information with children or other potential caregivers.

Nonetheless, there are numerous reasons why advance planning is important. Below is a list of benefits experienced by the caregiver and the older person when they engage in planning for the future:

- The care receiver and caregiver develop strategies to address possible future events.
- Family disagreements are lessened.
- The older person practices self-determination.
- Decisions are made without the added pressure of a crisis situation.
- The caregiver's task of making decisions for the older person is lessened.
- The older person's finances are put in order and bills are paid on time.
- Family resources are protected.

Advance planning is exactly what it states—planning in advance of a health care or other crisis. The aging person and potential caregivers get together to discuss how financial and health care decisions are to be made both now and in the future. Such planning involves anticipating future events and identifying ways to assure that assets are protected, the older person's decisions are respected, and the caregiver is able to execute solutions on behalf of the older person.

You might find that talking about these issues with your relative is very difficult, especially if this person questions your motives. Therefore, you must be reassuring when discussing legal and financial options. Let your relative know that your primary concern is to assure that she maintains decision-making authority and that you are able to carry out her wishes when she needs your assistance.

BEFORE YOU SPEND LOTS OF MONEY ON EXPERTS

At this point, you may be thinking, "Advance planning is a great idea but it is probably too expensive." In most instances, you will find that the expense involved in planning is minimal when compared to the security and peace of mind received. However, you do want to avoid unnecessary expenses for services that do not fit your situation. Before spending a lot of money on experts, consider the following tips:

✓ Sit down with your relative. Review the Legal, Financial, and Insurance section of your Care Log. Identify areas where you might need assistance. Realize that your circumstances may not warrant the attention of a professional.

✓ Review this chapter with your older relative. Discuss the legal and financial options that might be useful. Put your needs in writing. Be as specific as possible.

✓ For each need you have identified, make a list of questions that you would like to discuss with a professional. Again, be as specific as possible.

✓ Read, read, and read some more. Get copies of the materials listed at the end of this chapter. Order *Elder Care: Choosing and Financing Long Term Care* by Joseph Matthews from Nolo Press, 950 Parker Street, Berkeley, CA 94710, (415) 549-1976. This book costs $20.95 (including shipping) and covers health planning, estate planning, and insurance.

✓ Identify free or discounted legal and financial services. Ask family and friends who are lawyers, financial planners or insurance agents to give you their free expert opinion. Most professionals offer free initial consultation where they conduct a quick analysis of your situation. Each state provides free or discounted legal services for older people. Contact the local department on aging in your relative's city for further information. Also contact the local bar association to find out if they have any special programs for seniors.

✓ Identify at least three persons who specialize in areas in which you need assistance.

◊ Ask your family and friends for referrals.

◊ Ask your local bar association to refer attorneys who specialize in issues you are concerned about.

◊ Contact the National Academy of Elder Law Attorneys at 655 N. Alvernon Way #108, Tucson, AZ 85711, (602) 881-4005. The Academy can send you information on how to select an elder law attorney, a lawyer who specializes in concerns of seniors.

◊ Contact the National Insurance Consumers Helpline at (800) 942-4242 to get information on all types of insurance and referrals to other sources of information.

◊ Contact your local department on aging to identify health care counseling programs for seniors.

◊ Call the National Association of Personal Financial Advisors at (709) 537-7722 for a list of financial planners in your area.

✓ Interview each person. Make sure they have experience working with situations similar to yours. Ask if the person has received any special certifications or designations in the field. Ask for a list of references and contact each one. Compare fee structures and be aware of hidden costs. Ask what you can do to reduce your fee.

✓ Ask what is expected of you and what you should bring to the first official meeting.

By following these recommendations you will be able to figure out the type of professional you need and how to find them, what you want them to do, and how to prepare for your working relationship.

LEGAL OPTIONS

There are a number of legal options available to you and your relative that are quite useful for protecting assets and providing for future decision making. Following is an overview of legal arrangements that can be useful to caregivers. Again, you may want to consult an attorney to discuss your specific situation.

Will—A legal instrument whereby a person identifies who will receive his assets after his death. All caregivers and care receivers should have a will and all wills should be reviewed for accuracy every three years. When a person dies without a will, survivors are often faced with confusion and conflict.

Living Will —A legal document, recognized in 40 states and the District of Columbia, by which the older person specifies withholding of life support treatment if she is terminally ill. Living wills relieve caregivers from having to decide whether to administer or withhold life support treatments.

Power of Attorney—An instrument that gives someone else the authority to act on your behalf. In a caregiving situation, the older person can specify the responsibilities she gives to the caregiver. A basic power of attorney becomes invalid if the older person becomes incapacitated.

Springing Power of Attorney—A power of attorney that *goes into effect* only when the older person becomes incapacitated. The older person can specify how incapacity is defined and under what circumstances the power of attorney goes into effect. This instrument allows an older person to retain personal control until she is no longer able to do so.

Durable Power of Attorney—A power of attorney that goes into effect while a senior is healthy and *remains in effect* after the older person has become incapacitated. This instrument allows an older person to continue her decision-making plan while she is healthy or disabled.

Durable Power of Attorney for Health Care—A durable power of attorney that gives another person the authority to make health care decisions. To assure that the document is all inclusive, the older person and caregiver will want to specify preferences regarding all aspects of health treatment, including use of experimental drugs, resuscitation, intravenous nutrition, and use of life support equipment.

Trust—An estate planning document that allows an older person to transfer assets to a trust to benefit another person. Trusts help older persons pass on assets to caregivers so that the caregiver saves on estate taxes and avoids probate, a process of executing a will.

Irrevocable Trust—A trust that can not be changed once it is established.

Revocable Trust—A trust that can be changed.

FINANCIAL AND INSURANCE OPTIONS

In addition to legal instruments, there are also financial options available to simplify financial management and help finance long-term care. Again, you and your older relative are encouraged to seek out professionals who can help you find the options that best suit your situation.

Following is a brief description of financial options you and your older relative may want to consider.

Joint Ownership—A form of shared ownership by two or more persons. Accounts and assets held by "you (the caregiver) *and* your older relative" require both signatures for transactions. Accounts held by "you *or* your relative" require one signature for transactions. Caregivers are advised to consider how joint ownership will affect Medicaid eligibility and receipt of community resources before establishing joint ownership.

Representative Payee—A program that allows a caregiver to receive government benefit payments on behalf of an older person who is not capable of managing the payment. The Social Security Administration can provide further information on how a caregiver can become a representative payee.

Guardianship—A legal process whereby the courts give a caregiver authority to manage an older person's personal and/or financial affairs because the older person is no longer able to do so. State laws on guardianship vary tremendously. Further information can be obtained from a local law school or legal program for the elderly.

Supplemental Security Income—A federal payment for the blind and disabled of any age and low income elderly.

Medicare—A federal health insurance program for older Americans administered by the Social Security Administration. Part A covers hospital care and Part B covers doctors' fees. The Social Security Administration can answer any questions caregivers have regarding Medicare.

Qualified Medicare Beneficiary Program—A national program, administered by state and local departments of social services, that pays Medicare premiums, deductibles and coinsurance for persons with limited income and resources.

Medicaid—A federal/state health insurance program for low income elderly, and blind and disabled persons of any age. Medicaid covers home care and nursing home costs provided by eligible facilities for persons meeting the financial guidelines. Many times older persons "spend down" or deplete financial assets before becoming eligible for Medicaid. Eligibility guidelines vary from state to state, therefore caregivers should contact the Department of Human Services in their relative's area for specific information.

Medigap Policies—Medicare Supplemental Insurance, or "Medigap," is private insurance that pays the portion of medical bills not paid for by Medicare. Medigap policies only cover charges approved by Medicare as medically necessary. Caregivers will want to make sure that their older relative has only one Medigap policy as multiple policies offer the same coverage.

Long-Term Care Insurance—An insurance that provides financing for nursing home care and other long-term care services. These policies are useful to older persons who have substantial assets to protect. Policies vary greatly so caregivers are encouraged to contact several private insurance companies and compare policies.

FINANCIAL CONSIDERATIONS FOR CAREGIVERS

As a caregiver, you will probably spend your own money on care-related activities such as long distance telephone bills, travel expenses, paying for hired help, or purchasing supplies. In fact, a national survey of caregivers conducted by AARP indicates that caregivers spend an average of $117 per month on caregiving. Unfortunately, there are no provisions for long distance caregivers to be reimbursed for these expenses.

It is important that you set aside money to pay for these expenses if at all possible. This may be difficult for caregivers who have few reserves to meet current expenses. In such cases, it may be possible to persuade family members to donate a certain amount of money per month to pay for the care of your older relative. Having finances available will make your life much easier. It will allow you to travel, make long distance telephone calls, and purchase items without worrying about how you will pay the bills. Here is what Ron, a 44-year-old caregiver, had to say about organizing his finances to prepare for an emergency:

"I know I need to have some financial reserves to care for my parents. If there is an emergency, I can just pick up and fly 3,000 miles to be with them.

I have a travel emergency fund. I try to save as much as possible and I try not to accumulate a lot of bills. If my parents need me, I will be able to cover my travel expenses; and, in the event of a long term stay, I will use the money to cover my current responsibilities at home. I have a wife and children to help support. I keep 200 hours of annual leave so that I won't have to take time off without pay. It is very important to me to be able to be with my parents whenever they need me. It is equally as important to maintain the financial stability of my home."

Ron has done an excellent job preparing. During an actual emergency, he may find that he needs additional finances and that he will need to take time off work without pay. Nonetheless, he will be better able to deal with the financial costs associated with the emergency or the day to day expenses that can amount to a small fortune. That is why it is important for all caregivers to save.

DECISIONS, DECISIONS, DECISIONS

After reviewing this chapter, you may feel a little overwhelmed by the decisions to be made. Some of the options discussed above are appropriate for your situation while others are not. Before you spend money on attorneys, financial planners, or insurance agents, sit down with your older relative and go over all the options available. This will help define your goals and make it easier to talk to legal and financial experts when the time comes to do so. With a clear understanding of what you and your older relative need now and in the future, you will probably find that financial and legal decisions are not as difficult as they first appeared.

· · · · · · · · ·

This chapter provided highlights of the legal and financial options that can help you make decisions today and take charge of your future. In the next chapter, you will review the goals to be accomplished during your care commute.

TO DO IN THE NEXT TWO WEEKS

✓ Contact Concerns for Dying at 250 W. 57th Street, New York, NY 10107, (212) 246-6962, for advice and written information on durable power of attorney for health care.

✓ Contact the neighborhood legal services organization in your relative's area.

✓ Contact the local Bar Association in your relative's area to get several names of attorneys from the lawyer referral service.

✓ Order a free copy of the following resources from AARP Fulfillment, 601 E Street, NW, Washington, DC 20049: *Guide to Probate* (order #D13822); *Tomorrow's Choices: Preparing Now for Future Legal, Financial, and Health Care Decisions* (order #D13479); *Before You Buy: A Guide to Long Term Care Insurance* (order #D12893).

✓ Contact the Social Security Administration at (800) 772-1213 to have your relative's check deposited directly into a bank account to avoid having their check stolen.

✓ Write the local department of human services in your relative's area requesting information about Medicaid eligibility.

✓ Contact the Health Insurance Association of America at P.O. Box 41455, Washington, DC 20018 for a free copy of "A Consumer's Guide to Medicare Supplemental Insurance."

✓ Begin talking to your relative about financial and legal issues. Find out how she prefers matters to be handled if she is no longer able to make decisions.

Chapter Seven

SETTING AND ACCOMPLISHING MILESTONES

. . . .

"I simply didn't know where to start — it was obvious that my grandmother could no longer stay by herself. She had set the kitchen on fire, her neighbors complained that she would play the TV too loud during the night, and she hadn't paid her rent in two months. There was so much to do in such a short time. I didn't even know where to start. I felt terrible because I knew I made some decisions too quickly but I couldn't afford to be off work for very long."

—*Leslie Jean, computer programmer, age 49*

CARE PROVIDERS SELDOM DO ADVANCE PLANNING TO schedule their time during visits with their relative. Once they arrive at the older person's home, they panic and make hasty decisions. They feel completely stressed out during the trip, have little opportunity to share quality time with the older person, and feel guilty once they return home. As a caregiver, you may feel like Leslie Jean. Where do you start? How can you avoid making unwise decisions?

As the earlier chapters highlight, there are a number of tasks you can accomplish before your care commute. Nonetheless, there will still be a number of tasks to complete during your trip—perhaps too many. What can you realistically accomplish during a short trip?

This chapter goes a step further by helping you identify milestones that you can accomplish during your visit. It provides you with information on how to plan an extended weekend trip to your relative's home where important tasks can be accomplished. It discusses the three basic goals of any trip: assessment, care coordination, and setting up a monitoring system. By following the guidelines presented, you should be able to address areas of primary concern during your trip.

If possible, plan your trip around a weekend. This will give you more time to accomplish the responsibilities at hand while only taking three days off work. Plan to arrive at your relative's home on Friday evening. This will allow you some time to enjoy one another's company before the work begins. Commit Saturday and Sunday to confirming your initial assessment, verifying your top two priorities, meeting with your informal network, and locating needed documents before approaching the service system. On Monday and Tuesday, you can work with service providers and make sure a monitoring mechanism is in place that will allow you to check with others on the particulars of the elder's care from your home. Reserve Wednesday to tie up any loose ends and to travel back home.

BE REALISTIC

After reading the previous chapters, you may be feeling overwhelmed. Keep in mind that there are others who can help. Also, you must be realistic about how quickly you can address all of your concerns. Establishing a complete care plan takes time and may require more than one, five-day trip to your relative's home. In many cases, caregivers must deal with a series of different problems as their relative's needs change. Do not panic. Prioritize the issues of concern and deal with the most important concerns first.

ASSESSMENT

If you followed the examples outlined in chapter 2, you already have some idea of the primary needs of the older person. You have talked with the elder and members of your support network about issues of concern. You have also spoken to social service agencies and scheduled appointments. So when you arrive with your Care Log in hand, you already have a compass to guide your way.

Yet, it is important to further verify that the primary concerns you identified from a distance are indeed the primary areas of concern. To begin verifying your initial assessment of the elder's condition, first review the Assessment and the Medical Information sections of your Care Log. Second, observe, observe, observe! Become a master at observation. And remember that it is important to remain as objective as possible.

While verifying your initial assessment, be aware of the following:
- Are friends calling or stopping by to visit your relative?
- Is the house clean and in good repair? Are there safety concerns such as a loose bannister, cracked stairs, or leaking furnace?
- Is the older person able to drive or use some other mode of transportation?
- Is your relative well-groomed?
- Is there fresh food in the house? Are there leftovers? Is your relative able to cook easily?
- Are you aware of the older person's spiritual and emotional needs?

The next step is a family meeting. Contact other interested members of your family and schedule a meeting during your visit to discuss your relative's well being. A family meeting will allow you to discuss with the older person and other family members your impressions, review tasks completed, and strategize regarding the best approach to providing care. Ideally, a family meeting should take place face-to-face in the older person's home. Or, the meeting can be held on the telephone via a conference call. Contact an AT&T operator to get further information on how to set up a conference call.

Do not dwell on the fact that you may not be able to get all of your family members to cooperate. Realistically, a family meeting may not be possible for many families. There are numerous reasons why concerned family members are unable or unwilling to attend a family meeting.

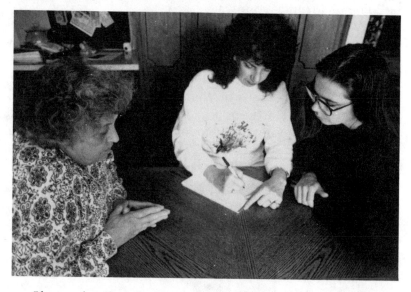

If your family is having a lot of difficulty communicating, you may want to solicit the assistance of a neutral third party. A family therapist or social worker may be able to facilitate a successful family meeting and help you with joint decision making. Sometimes, there are no other family members. In these cases, the caregiver and the elder will be responsible for setting and accomplishing the milestones addressed in this chapter.

For caregivers who are able to arrange a family meeting, send each member of your family a copy of the ground rules and a tentative agenda. Make sure someone agrees to take notes and distribute the minutes to all members within three weeks after the meeting. Ask everyone who will be attending to agree to the following:

- Everyone must agree with the goal of the meeting—to provide the senior with the assistance needed and to make sure that she can continue living as independently as possible.
- No one is blamed for past or current mistakes. The objective is to move on from this point.
- Everyone has a right to their own opinion, and their opinion must be listened to and respected by all parties.
- Everyone has the right to disagree and to voice opposing opinions in a calm, rational manner.
- Everyone present has an active voice in deciding how to best share in present and future tasks.
- If she is capable, the older person should be an active participant and retain ultimate decision-making authority, unless safety and health concerns are overriding issues.

It is important to bring all major concerns to the table and to reaffirm your top two priorities. Be sure to add to the list other topics that need discussing. This line of conversation may be difficult, but it is necessary.

Here are some subjects you should consider discussing even if you and your relative are the only two meeting:

- In what kinds of activities has the older person recently been involved? Does she ever feel lonely?
- Is housework manageable, including heavy cleaning?
- Is transportation a concern? When is transportation needed?
- Does the house or apartment meet the older person's needs? Is it too large or difficult to maintain?
- Is assistance needed with personal care like bathing, dressing, and grooming?
- Are nutritious meals being prepared and eaten?
- What are other important needs? (Make a list.)

CARE COORDINATION

Once you have come to some agreement about the most important needs, begin exploring how each of these needs can be addressed. Be sure to begin with your top two concerns and continue addressing as many issues as possible in order of importance. Remember, each family member present should take responsibility for dealing with specific areas of concern. Use the Informal Network section of your Care Log to list each individual's commitment.

For areas of concern that are not addressed by the family, turn to the other members of your informal network for assistance. Explore how these people can assist you. If at this point you still have unmet concerns, solicit help from the health or social services agencies in your relative's community.

In pulling together a care plan or a strategy for providing care, your primary goal is to assure that every problem is met in a coordinated fashion. Your family, friends, and service providers should understand what they are supposed to do and when the task should be completed. It is important to make sure that no one's responsibility overlaps with that of another person. You want all of your helpers to feel useful.

SETTING UP A MONITORING SYSTEM

Once you have a care plan in place, you will want to set up a process whereby you can monitor your relative's condition and care from a distance. Start by contacting everyone involved and reiterate what each person or organization has agreed to do. This is an important step because it allows you to make sure that your understanding of the support to be given is accurate.

Again, let your support network know that you appreciate the help given and that you would like to be able to call them to find out how things are going. Let them know how often you plan to contact them. For the first month or two, you may want to call them every two weeks. When you feel comfortable with your care plan, you may want to decrease your calls to once every four to six weeks. Make sure they have your telephone number in case of emergency or if they are no longer able to provide assistance. Explain that they can call you collect. The objective is to be able to leave your relative knowing exactly what needs are being addressed and by whom. Also, you have begun establishing a healthy rapport with members of your support network and you have expressed appreciation for their involvement.

The following example shows how Caryn used a five-day visit with her father to gather the information she needed to set up an effective monitoring system:

Friday
—Visit Dad, explain my plans for the balance of the trip.
—Observe the conditions of the house, particularly indication of Dad's nutritional habits.
—Call my sister, Gwen, to confirm the family meeting.
—Start contacting members of the informal network.

Saturday
—Complete the assessment.
—Sit down with Dad and Gwen and prioritize Dad's needs.
—Review with Dad and Gwen the legal and financial issues outlined in chapter 6 of *Long Distance Caregiving*.
—Continue talking with the informal network about options for care. Verify the assistance they are willing to provide and find assistance in areas not covered by my network.
—Update the Informal Resources section of the Care Log.
—Review information received from social service agencies.
—Complete the applications I received in the mail from service agencies.

Sunday
—Complete work begun on Saturday.
—Begin locating needed documents and make copies.
—Update the Community Resources section in my Care Log by listing individual needs followed by the name, address, and telephone of agencies that can meet those needs.
—Make a list of questions to ask each service provider such as the nature of the service, application process, fees, and how the program is reviewed for quality.

Monday
—Start calling service providers at 9 a.m. Gather as much information as possible. Explain that I live out of town. Schedule a meeting for that afternoon or the following day.
—If possible, take Dad along on my appointments with service providers. Also take any needed documents and my Care Log.
—Complete necessary paperwork.

Tuesday
—Continue meeting with service providers.
—Select the type of service that best meets Dad's needs. Select an agency to address each of Dad's primary needs if I have not already done so.
—Create a "Resources in Place" page under the Community Resources section of my Care Log. List each area of need and the resource in place to address each concern. Make a copy for Dad and interested family members.
—Call all resources in place to thank them for their help.
—Set up a monitoring procedure.

Wednesday
—Complete unfinished business.
—Travel home.

· · · · · · · · ·

In this chapter you were shown how to schedule a productive five-day visit with your older relative. You were provided with tips for conducting an assessment of your relative's needs, how to run a family meeting, how to organize for meetings with community agencies, and how to monitor your care plan from a distance. The next chapter focuses on what you can do when your care plan needs to be fine-tuned.

TO DO IN THE NEXT TWO WEEKS

✓ Contact your family and share your plans for assisting the older person.

✓ Schedule a date for the family meeting.

✓ Send an agenda and a copy of the ground rules for the family meeting to each person planning to attend.

✓ Talk with your local department on aging to gather tips for dealing with "aging network" agencies that work with elderly persons and their family caregivers.

✓ Develop a schedule of tasks to complete and people to meet during your visit.

Chapter Eight

ADJUSTING YOUR CARE PLAN

. . . .

"It never fails. I'd spend days at my Mom's place arranging for people to help take care of her. A few days later, I'd get a call—she wouldn't let anybody in the house. When I call her, she swears that no one came to the house or that she couldn't see who was at the door, or she didn't open the door because she thought it was a salesperson. Then I'd have to drive two-and-a-half hours to her house, explain the same things over and over and beg the homecare worker and the church volunteer to come back again. No matter what I do, Mom refuses to accept help."

—*Joyce, secretary, age 48*

AS A LONG DISTANCE CAREGIVER, YOU MAY FIND THAT YOUR care coordination skills are frequently being put to the test, and that your Care Log has become your constant companion. But even if you have followed the steps in the first few chapters to the letter, you may still find that your plan of care is not working as well as you had hoped: your relative could refuse to accept care, as is the case of Joyce; your helpers may be unreliable or unsuitable; your relative's needs may change; or an emergency can arise. In any case, it is important to be sure that your monitoring system works adequately so that you are alerted when your relative's care plan needs to be fine-tuned. The purpose of this chapter is to show you ways to monitor and alter your care plan when it becomes necessary.

THE MONITORING SYSTEM

Chapter 3 discussed how to set up a monitoring system for your support network and chapter 5 focused on monitoring the social service system. These two chapters highlight the importance of making sure that you, your relative, and anyone else involved in providing help are clear about the assistance to be given. Each party has your telephone number and mailing address and everyone has been instructed to contact you should a problem arise.

Once you have this system in place, take the lead in establishing how the system will work. You may be disappointed if you wait for members of your support network to contact you on a regular basis. You will want to write or telephone them regularly to establish a pattern of communication and good rapport. About three to four weeks after your care commute, talk with your relative about the care plan. Find out if it is working to your relative's satisfaction. Make sure services are being delivered according to the agreed-upon schedule. Make note of any concerns your relative may have and decide how to best address these concerns. Some matters can be handled by your relative, but you will have to intervene to resolve some concerns.

Turn to the "Resources in Place" page in the Community Resources section of your Care Log. Select your key contact persons and place a star by their names. (Key contacts are persons who are delivering a vital service, persons who are truly interested in your relative's well-being, or simply people who visit your relative on a regular basis.) Key contact persons should be the first to know when something is going wrong. By selecting key contacts, you eliminate the need to call numerous members of your support network.

Call your key contact people and persons with whom your relative has expressed concern. Express your gratitude for their assistance (remember, you can not say thank-you too much to members of your support network). Talk with each key contact person about the following issues:

- Explain that you would like to call and/or write them from time to time to make sure that everything is ok.
- Find out when they last saw your relative. What were their general impressions of your relative's well-being?
- Discuss issues that concern you or your relative.
- Discuss their reactions to providing care. Reconfirm their willingness to help.
- If payment for services is required, confirm the fee and how payments are to be made.
- Ask them to drop you a note from time to time to let you know how things are going.
- Remind them to call you collect, immediately, if they feel there is a problem or concern you need to know about.

After this initial contact, you may want to speak with your key contacts every four to six weeks, or more often if the need arises. It is important to establish a pattern of regular contact in order to establish a good rapport. If conversations are planned in advance they need not be long.

Although you have established a pattern to monitor your support system, there will be times when unexpected problems arise. Your system of care will need modification for a number of reasons. Following are some of the more common issues that will cause you to adjust your care plan. Also included are tips to resolve these issues.

YOUR RELATIVE REFUSES HELP

There may be times when your relative does not want any assistance and refuses to cooperate with helpers. It is important to understand why the person rejects help. Following is a list of reasons why some elders do not accept help from others:

- Seniors sometimes feel that accepting help is an admission of dependency.
- Some elders regard accepting services as a form of welfare.
- Your relative may be concerned about the cost of the service.

- Your relative may want you, and not someone else, to deliver the care needed.
- The older person might be afraid of strangers, particularly if they must come to the home to deliver the service.
- The person delivering care may be unacceptable to the older person.

Once you know why your relative is refusing assistance, you can develop strategies to encourage her to accept help. Everyone wants to feel able to take care of themselves and control their own destiny. Overcoming feelings of dependency · is tough. Perhaps one way to help elders deal with these feelings is to focus on how accepting help in one area will help them function independently in another area. For example, Erica explained to her mother that she was no longer able to keep her house clean and therefore someone else was going to help her with the housework. She explained further that her mother (who dearly loved bridge) would not be able to continue having bridge parties in a dirty house.

Some older persons feel that social services are either a form of welfare or are too expensive. In the first case, you will want to explain that these services are paid for by their tax dollars and that every older person in America has the right to utilize senior services. You can also encourage her to give donations to service agencies if that would make her feel better. If your relative is concerned about the expense of the service, tell her that you want to give the service as a present or explain how she can budget her money to pay for the service.

Concerns about who delivers services are common. Some elders feel that the caregiver is the only one who should give them help. Or, perhaps the fear of strangers is so intense that the older person will not allow others to help. In these situations, caregivers must appeal to reason by explaining why they are unable to provide care. They must find ways to make strangers more acceptable. One way is to ask someone whom the older person trusts, such as a minister or rabbi, or close freind or social worker, to recommend a care provider. A personal reference may be all that is needed. Or you may want to ask someone the older person trusts to be on hand when the "stranger" is present. This may make the older person feel more comfortable.

Keep in mind that there may be situations when no matter how loving and kind a worker is, the older person will still find them unacceptable. This may be due to racial or ethnic differences, the age of the worker, language barriers, the appearance of the helper, or a number of other factors. If this is the case with your relative, there may not be much you can do other than encouraging the older person to accept differences in people and insisting that your relative allow the helper to do her job.

There are times, however, when an older person is justified in refusing help. Unfortunately, some people who are supposedly helping elders are actually abusing them. If your relative accuses a helper of abuse, this accusation should be investigated carefully. You, or possibly someone from your support network, will want to talk with the care provider to try to resolve the conflict; or speak with the provider's supervisor if she is a paid employee. Perhaps someone from the support network would be willing to investigate the matter. If accusations are grounded, the helper should be dismissed immediately. If this person is connected to an agency, you will want to make a formal complaint and seek retribution if necessary.

UNRELIABLE HELP

Your care plan may also break down because the service provider is unreliable. You may find that helpers do not show up on time or sometimes do not show up at all. And even when they are with your relative, they may not complete tasks to your satisfaction. It does not matter whether you are paying for this assistance or not, members of your support network should be responsive and responsible.

When you are faced with unreliable help, decide who will deal with the matter—you, your relative, or someone else from your support network. Following are a few problem-solving techniques that both you and your relative might find helpful:

- *Clearly identify your dissatisfaction.* Chapters 4 and 7 suggest that you send a copy of your expectations to each member of your support network. If you followed this advice, you can easily write down your concerns.
- *Discuss your concerns with the care provider.* Begin your discussion in a nonthreatening manner. Start with compliments and then explain your expectations. Check to see if the care provider has a similar understanding of her job responsibilities. If you do not have the same understanding, renegotiate until you come to an agreement. If your helper agrees with your expectations, explain why you feel your expectations have not been met and provide concrete examples of why you are dissatisfied.
- *Agree to a trial period.* Once you have come to an agreement about how the service will be delivered, suggest that you take the next 30 days to work together under the new agreement. You may want to put this agreement in writing and share a copy with the care provider.
- *Revisit the issues.* After 30 days, re-evaluate the situation. If you can see improvement, express your appreciation. If you are still not satisfied, you may need to look for someone else to assist you. If your helper is a paid care provider, discuss your concerns with their supervisor.
- *Contact the supervisor.* Give thought to how you would like to resolve your concerns before calling the supervisor. Think about whether you want another worker, a discount, or more direct supervision of the worker. Clearly discuss your concerns with the supervisor and try to come to a mutual agreement as to how the matter might be rectified.
- *Establish a trial period.* Take 30 days to review the solution you are implementing with the supervisor. If the solution works well, notify the supervisor. If it doesn't, locate another service provider and dismiss the current worker.

Of course, there are instances when you do not have time to go through this long process. If at any time the older person's health or well-being is in jeopardy, discontinue a service and begin looking for alternatives. Depending on the severity of your complaint, you may also want to report the incident to the proper oversight agency.

NEEDS CHANGE OVER TIME

The needs of the older person will change over time. This is one of the reasons it is important to establish rapport with your support network—especially with your key contact persons—so that they can keep you informed of changes. Your care plan will need to be adjusted as the needs of the older person change. Adding to your existing care plan is much easier than developing a new plan. Contact the sources of information listed in your Care Log and ask them to suggest services that will meet current needs. If you have a good list of information sources to draw from, you may not need to visit your relative's home in order to modify the care plan.

IF AN EMERGENCY OCCURS

If an emergency or sudden illness occurs, it is obvious that you will need to make some quick adjustments to your care plan. New services may be needed and old services may need to be canceled. Chapter 3 will help you decide whether you can postpone a trip or not. If you decide you must travel to your relative's home, remember to take your Care Log. It will help you identify programs and services to meet your current and future needs.

. . . .

This chapter focused on circumstances that will cause you to adjust your care plan. You were also provided tips for making needed adjustments. The next chapter covers issues to consider when your relative needs to move to more suitable housing.

TO DO IN THE NEXT TWO WEEKS

✓ Identify key contact persons.

✓ Develop a schedule of how often you will telephone or write notes to your key contact persons. Place this information on a calendar for quick and easy reference.

✓ Check in with other interested family members.

✓ Compose your thoughts to convince your older relative to accept help from others.

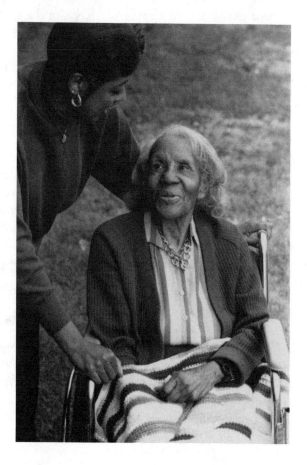

Chapter Nine

RELOCATION
When, Who, and Where

·· · · · · · · ·

"My concern about relocation is having a mother who really likes her house. How do I know when she needs to leave her house? And how do I help her accept the idea of having to live with other people in some kind of facility — whether it is a community residential facility or a nursing home? How do I deal with my sense of letting her down?"

—Barbara, management consultant, age 47

BARBARA'S FEELINGS AND QUESTIONS ARE TYPICAL. CARE-givers struggle with these issues because there are no clear barometers that show when relocation is best for all persons involved. All too often caregivers panic, fearing that their older relative cannot live alone when all that is needed is a simple modification to the home and a couple of community services. On the other hand, family members feel remorse if the older person becomes ill or has an accident that could have been avoided had the older person moved to a more supportive environment.

When caregivers discuss the need to move an elder, they frequently focus on nursing home placement or combining households with the older person. Often, neither the caregiver nor the older person are familiar with the various housing choices that offer different levels of support. They therefore do not have enough information to select the best alternative.

There are several issues to review and understand before making changes in the current living arrangements. This chapter will discuss the when, who, and where issues of relocation. You will explore issues to consider in deciding who needs to relocate and when the move is appropriate. You will examine different housing options and explore whether combining households with your elder relative is realistic. And, you will review tips to help your relative adjust to the new living arrangement.

RELOCATION—WHEN

Relocating is hard for older persons. The decision to move can be a very emotional and stressful life event. Their home often provides a sense of independence, familiarity and connectedness to the community. Most elders do not want to leave their homes and most certainly do not want to live with adult children. In fact, research shows that older persons prefer to stay in their own homes for as long as possible. Therefore, you will want to investigate services to keep the older person in the home before considering a different living arrangement.

It is difficult to know when an older person's needs are best met in a more supportive environment. Often it is a matter of opinion. And remember, your opinions may differ from those of your relative. Caregivers must learn to balance their relative's wishes to remain independent with issues of concern and safety. Clearly, however, the following situations suggest that housing adjustments are needed:

- A physician or other health care professional recommends a change in the current housing arrangement.
- The older person needs care or supervision 24 hours a day due to mental or physical limitations.
- Concrete evidence suggests that the safety of the older person is at risk.
- The elder can no longer move around in the current home due to structural barriers or physical impairments.

- The current home does not meet fire, health, or safety standards.
- The neighborhood has deteriorated and is unsafe.

If you suspect that your relative needs another type of housing, solicit input from your key contact persons. Ask them if they have noticed that the house needs a thorough cleaning or repair. Are there any safety or health hazards in the home? Can your relative move around freely? Review the Assessment section of your Care Log. Have your relative's abilities changed?

If possible, visit your relative's home immediately if you suspect that their health, safety or welfare is in jeopardy. The following suggestions will help you talk with your relative concerning their need to relocate:

- Keep in mind that this may be a very sensitive topic for your relative. Be as tactful as possible in discussing your observations and fears.
- Listen to your relative. Ask them for suggestions to address your concerns.
- Review all possible alternatives. What does your relative need in order to remain in the home? Should you combine households? What types of housing are available to meet your relative's needs?
- Visit various housing alternatives with your relative.
- Allow your relative to select the least restrictive setting.
- When possible, consider your decision for a trial period of 60 days. You can explore other options if the first one is not suitable.

RELOCATION—WHO

If you and your relative conclude that caregiving would be easier if you were geographically closer, the next logical question is who is going to move, you or your relative. There are a number of advantages and disadvantages to either decision. The following questions will help you and your relative begin discussing who should relocate. As your conversation continues, you will uncover specific issues pertaining to your situation that deserve consideration.

- Will you need to, and be able to, secure employment in your relative's community?
- How much will it cost to move?
- Would the move result in an increase or decrease in living expenses?
- Will you or your relative be able to pursue the social, recreational, and educational activities you currently enjoy?
- How would the move affect other family members?
- Will you have family, friends, and agencies available to help you with caregiving activities? Review the Informal Support and Resources sections of your Care Log.
- Where will you live?
- How would your decision not to move affect your relative's condition?

If you are honest in considering these questions and the complexities of your situation, you will be able to make a rational decision about who should move. In some cases, you may find that relocation is not possible or desirable for either you or your relative.

RELOCATION—WHERE

When you discover that your older relative's housing is inappropriate, remember there are a number of housing options to consider. If your relative is in fairly good physical and mental health, then relocation may be simply a matter of moving to a smaller home. Your options in this case include a small house, a condominium, a cooperative, or an apartment. Each option presents a different set of financial obligations, responsibilities, and tax considerations. You might consider speaking with a local real estate management company to discuss the advantages and disadvantages of these options.

In most caregiving situations, however, the topic of relocation arises because the older person is experiencing some limitations that make it difficult for her to live alone without support.

If this is your experience, start by reviewing the Community Resources section of your Care Log and the directory of services from your relative's community. Consider using community resources to help the older person remain at home.

If you do not already have information on senior housing, contact the local department on aging and the National Elder-care Institute on Housing at the University of Southern California, Andrus Gerontology Center, Los Angeles, CA 90089, (213) 740-1364. Have them send you copies of any information they have on senior housing alternatives. Make notations about housing options under the Resources section of your Care Log.

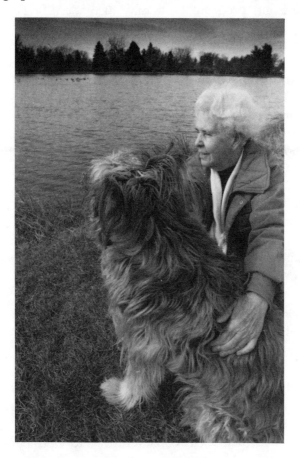

You and your relative will want to consider the following housing options. While you are reviewing possibilities, keep in mind that the primary goals are to provide the support needed and to protect independence.

House Sharing

Your relative may be able to share a house with someone who agrees to provide assistance in exchange for discounted or free room and board. There are shared housing projects that can match your relative with potential housemates. Contact the local department on aging to locate shared housing programs. If there is no program, you may also identify housemates through a local church, university or senior center.

Another housing sharing option is for the caregiver to combine households with the older person. Many caregivers feel it would be easier to share a household with their older relative. In reality, this is not always the case. And once someone has moved to a different town or state, it is not so easy to move back. Before combining households, you will need to think about how this decision will affect you, your relative, your spouse, and other family members.

Following is a list of considerations for persons thinking about combining households with an older relative:

- Are you and your relative able to live under the same roof? Strained relationships do not change because your relative needs your help.
- Is there adequate space for the two of you to combine households?
- What furniture will be stored or discarded?
- How will you protect one another's privacy?
- How will your day-to-day activities change?
- What are the best sleeping arrangements? Who will need to give up space to accommodate an extra person moving into the house?
- What are the financial considerations for both parties?
- Are community resources available?

- How will other family members assist with caregiving?
- Will you have sufficient time for your spouse and children?

Echo Housing and Accessory Apartments

Echo housing and accessory apartments are ideal for many caregivers and care receivers. Both types of housing provide complete privacy and the security of knowing that family is within walking distance. An echo house is a small, temporary house built in the back or on the side of a main home. An accessory apartment is a private apartment within the structure of a single-family home. Typically, the apartment is a complete, self-contained unit with a separate entrance. Older persons and caregivers considering either an echo house or accessory apartment may need to work with the local zoning board to get permits for such housing.

A good source of information on echo housing and accessory apartments is the American Association of Retired Persons (AARP). Write AARP's Membership Services Department at 601 E Street, NW, Washington, DC 20049 and ask for packet H0953 for information on echo housing and packet H0958 for information on accessory apartments.

Supportive Community Housing

There are a number of housing options available in the community that offer seniors various types of support. You and your older relative will want to identify the type of housing that best meets your needs and then visit several units. When evaluating the different types of supportive housing, keep in mind the following issues:
- Is the unit affordable?
- What services are included in the monthly rate?
- Can the older person bring in furniture and other personal belongings?
- Can the older person live with the rules and regulations?
- What are the staff's qualifications?
- Is the unit handicap accessible?

- Does the neighborhood appear safe? Are there stores, places to worship, businesses and services in close proximity?
- Is public transportation available?
- Are current residents satisfied?

Retirement Communities

Retirement communities are self-contained housing facilities that offer an array of recreational activities and some limited social services. Independent elders often select this type of housing. Typically, few provisions are available to the older person who becomes ill while living in a retirement community.

Continuing Care Retirement Communities (CCRCs)

CCRCs, or life care communities, offer older persons different levels of care. CCRCs provide recreational facilities, personal care services, support services, health care and medical care within the same setting. CCRCs require residents to pay a one-time entrance fee and monthly fees.

Congregate Housing

Congregate housing provides independent living space and limited services to elderly and disabled persons. These facilities vary from location to location but typically offer seniors one meal a day, recreational activities, and sometimes the services of a social worker. Residents living in congregate housing do not need 24-hour care. Most residents can function independently but like the idea of support at a distance. Many units are funded by the federal government and cater to moderate and low income elders.

Community Residential Facilities

Community residential facilities (also known as board and care homes, foster homes, and assisted living facilities) are appropriate for elders who need 24-hour supervision. Often, these facilities are large private homes with several seniors sharing common space. Some facilities are licensed by the state while others are not. These facilities offer services such as a room, assistance with personal care, meals, medications management, and laundry services.

Nursing Homes

For most caregivers, the thought of "putting their older relative in a nursing home" is depressing. For many, placing a parent in a nursing home represents failure as a caregiver. Likewise, many older persons resist nursing home placement feeling that it is the place where people go to die.

Despite the negative publicity nursing homes have received, many of them provide excellent care for elders who need 24-hour nursing services or supervision. Nursing homes provide meals, laundry, personal care, recreation, nursing services, administration of medications and therapies. Caregivers should work with the ombudsman at the local department on aging to carefully select a nursing home that provides quality care. An ombudsman is the person who investigates consumer complaints about community residential facilities and nursing homes. Ombudsmen are typically located in the office on aging.

ADJUSTING TO THE MOVE

If you or your relative decide to move, be realistic, be patient. The person who moves will long for their familiar home, furnishings, neighborhood, neighbors, etc. This is a normal reaction to change. It will take time to adjust to new surroundings. For some, the adjustment will be made quickly; but for others, the adjustment may be long and difficult.

If the older person is the one who decides to move, you will want to be supportive. As a caregiver, you can set the tone for the move. When possible, get the whole family involved. Constantly reenforce the benefits of the move and highlight the positive features of the new home. Help your relative select items to be discarded and donate them to a worthy charity. Ask that the organization send your relative a personalized thank-you note for the donation.

After the move, help your relative decorate the new home. Sponsor a family open house to get other relatives involved.

Visit as often as possible to help your relative become a part of the community. Explore the new location with your relative. Identify places to shop, churches and recreational facilities. Introduce your relative to neighbors and others in the community. Ask members of your support network to visit frequently.

. . . .

In this chapter, you learned about relocation issues. You were provided suggestions to help you decide whether it is best for you or your relative to relocate. You received guidance regarding when an older person needs to move to a more supportive environment. And, you received an overview of housing options. In the next chapter, you will learn about the very challenging situation of trying to care for your relative when you live in different countries.

THINGS TO DO IN THE NEXT TWO WEEKS

✓ Ask a member of your support network to give you an up-to-date report on your relative's well-being.

✓ Order information on senior housing from the local department on aging in your relative's community.

✓ If your relative is considering moving to your community, order information on housing from your local department on aging.

✓ Order a free copy of *Encountering Problems in Nursing Homes* (D13717) and *The Nursing Home Regulatory System* (D13716) from AARP Fulfillment, 601 E Street, NW, Washington, DC 20049.

✓ Talk with family members about various housing options.

Chapter Ten

CARING FROM
ANOTHER COUNTRY

· · · · · · · · ·

"When my grandmother got sick in Germany, we needed to decide quickly who could go to be with her, who had the most flexibility. We also had to make sure that things were taken care of at home. We had to stop the mail and the newspaper, review our bills, dispose of foods that would spoil while we were away and think about funeral arrangements, just in case. Inevitably, we needed to stay longer than we had originally planned."

—*Ulrike, consultant, age 28*

IF CAREGIVING FROM A DISTANT CITY OR STATE IS PERPLEXING, then caregiving from another country can only be described as totally bewildering. The distance involved in international caregiving poses serious challenges. It can result in unscheduled time away from work, extensive travel, huge telephone bills, and utter confusion. The physical stress of getting to one's relative is quite exhausting. Those who are unable to travel immediately may incur mammoth telephone bills. And caregivers who cannot travel to be by their relative's side experience tremendous remorse and other difficult emotions.

There are few hard and fast rules concerning international caregiving. Many circumstances determine the resources available to you and your relative. Local services in your relative's community, family and friends, and your financial reserves are all important factors. Knowing what to do and where to start is hard because the health care and service systems in other countries are very different from those in the United States. Some countries have an organized and effective system to care for seniors while others do not have any system.

This chapter helps you react to international caregiving situations. It provides useful tips and reviews valuable resources to help you respond to emergency situations. It also reviews issues you and your relative need to consider before either of you moves to another country or relocates to combine households.

BEFORE MOVING ABROAD

If either you or your older relative is thinking about moving to a foreign country, and you are a potential caregiver, the following items are issues you will want to discuss before the move:

- Review the Legal, Financial, and Insurance section of your Care Log. Make sure all documents are accessible and up-to-date.
- Insurance—What kind of health insurance provisions has your older relative made? Medicare does not cover hospital or medical services delivered in another country. Discuss the appropriate response should the person living abroad die. Consider purchasing insurance to pay for local burial or transporting that person's remains back to America.
- Legal protection—Make sure all needed legal documents are available, up-to-date and easy for you to use. The person moving abroad should execute two wills — one to dispose of assets in the United States and the other to dispose of assets in the country of residence.
- Purchase a medical alert bracelet. This bracelet will alert health workers of any medical problems, allergies, or reactions to medicine.
- Services for seniors—Make sure your relative understands the services he or she will receive from their country of

residence. It is also important to understand the types of services you can purchase and the cost of these services.

- Government benefits—Find out how to transfer benefit checks overseas by contacting the federal or state agency that issues the check.
- Discuss how you should respond to emergencies. You may want to write this information under the Miscellaneous section of your Care Log instead of relying on your memory. Apply for a passport just in case you need to travel to care for your relative.

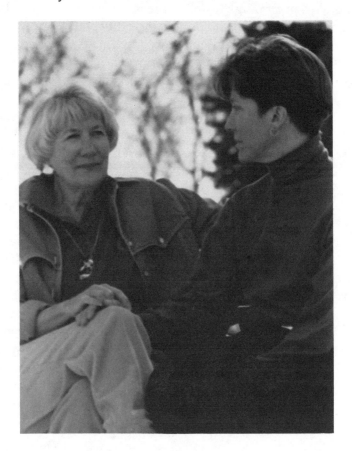

IMPORTANCE OF INFORMAL SUPPORT

Your informal support network is invaluable when international borders separate you from your older relative. Family and friends living near your relative are your first resource. In some instances, they are your only resource. They will be able to keep you abreast of the situation and serve as intermediaries between you and persons providing care to your relative. Therefore, keeping in touch with these people is very important.

Communicating with your relative and informal support network may range from simple to nearly impossible depending on the financial and political stability of the countries where you both live. The following tips will help you communicate effectively with your support network.

- Keep the informal support section of your Care Log up-to-date.
- Stay in contact with your support network at least once a month.
- Ask someone from your support network to help you identify resource organizations. Ask them to send you the names, addresses, and telephone numbers for the nearest health facilities, Red Cross or Red Crescent organization, and service providers. Ask them to send you written information (in English if possible) describing programs and services for seniors. Put this information in the Resources section of your Care Log.
- If necessary, pay key contact persons to provide incentive for their support.
- Make sure these persons understand the best way to stay in contact with you. Decide on the most effective and realistic method of communication, whether it be by telephone, letter, telegram, or through an international organization.
- If necessary, send your primary contact person money so he or she can contact you immediately should the need arise.

In addition to family and friends, it is also important to learn about resource organizations that can facilitate communication with your relative and help you respond to emergencies. The following information will help you understand the assistance you can expect depending on your circumstances. Keep in mind that in more developed parts of the world there may be several supports available, while in less developed countries there may be very few.

ASSISTANCE FOR MILITARY FAMILIES

Caregivers who are members of the United States Armed Forces have excellent communication resources. In addition, they are entitled to travel aid. These resources are available to military families no matter where they live in the world.

If you are in the military and your relative is experiencing an emergency situation, your family and friends can contact you through their local Red Cross chapter. The Red Cross will verify the situation and forward a message to your military base. Your commanding officer will notify you. You may then communicate back and forth through the Red Cross to check on the situation.

If the situation demands your presence, the Red Cross will request that you receive leave from your duties. If needed, you may apply for a no-interest loan to finance a trip to where your older relative lives. Once you arrive in your relative's city, the local Red Cross will help you arrange for the ongoing care of your relative by providing referrals to service organizations. In addition, Military Aid Societies may provide limited financial assistance. Although neither the Red Cross nor Military Aid Societies will provide long-term help, they are valuable resources for responding to short-term emergency situations.

ASSISTANCE FOR U.S. CITIZENS LIVING OVERSEAS

There are about two million Americans living abroad. Americans living abroad should register with the nearest U.S. embassy or consulate immediately after arrival. U.S. consular officers and agents, located at many service posts in foreign cities, are responsible for aiding Americans traveling or living abroad. Primary consular services include help with medical, legal, and financial difficulties. Other useful services include locating local service providers and transferring government benefits. Consular officers will help families arrange for local funerals or transport deceased persons back to the United States.

If your relative living abroad has a medical or emergency situation that needs your attention, a consular officer or agent may contact you. This person will facilitate communication with your older relative, tell you about local services, and help you transfer money to your relative. If your relative has signed a release of information form, they will keep you informed about the person's welfare.

If you cannot contact your older relative living abroad and you suspect that there is a problem, call the Citizen's Emergency Center of the State Department at (202) 647-5225 or (202) 634-3600. The Center deals with emergencies involving Americans in foreign countries. The Center's staff will work with consular staff to locate your relative and assess their welfare. You will receive a report if your relative has signed a release of information form. They also can assist in the return of an ill relative back to the United States.

ASSISTANCE FOR FOREIGN NATIONALS

Caregivers living in the United States who have relatives who are citizens of another country have few resources available to them. The lack of support is due to privacy laws in other countries and the inability of American organizations to interfere in the affairs of foreign nationals. (Foreign nationals are citizens of other countries.)

If this is your situation, your informal network is integral. Family, friends, and community members may be, in many instances, your only link to the older person. You will want to contact the embassy or consulate of the government where your relative lives. They can provide information on how the country operates and the resources that are available.

As a last resort, you may want to contact your local Red Cross chapter. There are about 150 Red Cross societies around the world. As each society operates differently, the type of assistance they can provide varies tremendously. In some cases, the Red Cross may be able to help you communicate with your relative.

RELOCATION ON THE INTERNATIONAL LEVEL

Chapter 9 reviews issues to consider before combining households with your older relative. In addition, there are other matters to consider before you or your relative move to another country in order to live together. Moving to another country is difficult for anyone because such a move involves a total readjustment of lifestyle. An international move is particularly challenging for older people who have had little or no experience with other cultures.

Relocating to the United States

Following are some questions you and your older relative will want to consider before moving to America:

- Is the older person physically able to make the trip?
- Will moving cause your relative intense loneliness?
- Is the older person able to speak and understand English?
- How will relocating affect retirement income?
- Will your relative's health insurance cover treatment in this country? If not, how will you pay for health expenses?
- Will you or someone else have the time to introduce your relative to life in America?
- How will you ensure that the older person has access to cultural activities and familiar foods?
- Can you introduce the older person to a peer from her homeland?

If you and your relative agree that she needs to move to the United States, test this arrangement for three to six months before making a permanent move. Contact the local office of the U.S. Immigration Service for the latest information on immigration regulations. Look in the government section of your telephone book to find your local office.

Generally, your relative can move to the U.S. either permanently or for medical treatment. If you are a U.S. citizen, you can petition for a spouse, child, adult son or daughter, or parent to immigrate to this country for permanent residence. A United States citizen is someone who was born in the U.S., a person born of U.S. citizens living outside of the country, or naturalized persons. A naturalized citizen is a foreign-born person who has lived in this country for five years or more and who has applied for and been accepted to become a citizen. There are no annual limits on the number of persons who can immigrate under this status. A citizen may also partition to bring a sibling to America. However, be aware that applications are currently being processed that were filed several years ago. Permanent residents may only partition to bring a spouse, child, or unmarried adult son or daughter to this country. A permanent resident is a non-citizen who has been granted the right to live in this country. There is no provision for a citizen or a permanent resident to sponsor a grandparent, older aunt or uncle, or stepparent for immigration.

If you want to bring your relative to the United States for medical treatment, obtain a statement from a U.S. medical facility that verifies their willingness to provide care and your obligation to pay for the services rendered. Mail this statement to your relative and have her take it to the U.S. consulate. The consulate may require additional documentation before issuing your relative a visa to visit the United States.

Relocating to Another Country

Before you decide to relocate to another country, consider the following questions:

- How stable is the country?
- What are the tax implications?
- How will you find employment if you want or need to work? How will you support yourself before you find employment?

- Do you speak the language and understand the customs of the country?
- Are you truly willing to change your life by moving to another country?

. . . .

This chapter provided you with valuable information for handling emergency situations when you are separated from your relative by international borders. It outlined steps to take before you or your relative move to another country. You were given a number of issues to consider if you are thinking about relocating to make caregiving easier. Hopefully, this information has helped you understand and prepare for international caregiving.

THINGS TO DO TWO MONTHS BEFORE YOUR OLDER RELATIVE MOVES ABROAD

✓ Get a medical statement from the older person's physician listing all medical conditions, prescription drugs, and the generic names of prescribed medicines. Keep a copy in the Medical Information section of your Care Log.

✓ Apply for your passport in case you need to travel suddenly. Passports are obtained from a passport agency, a local post office, or a federal or state court that accepts passport applications.

✓ Review your relative's health insurance policy to find out if it covers medical services delivered abroad. If not, contact your local insurance commissioner to identify companies offering this coverage.

✓ Call several airlines that fly to the country where your relative is moving to get the average cost for a round-trip ticket. Enter this information in the Travel section of your Care Log.

✓ Start saving money to cover the cost of your flight and one month's living expenses.

✓ Purchase as a present for your relative, *How To Stay Healthy While Traveling: A Guide for Today's World Traveler* by Bob Young, MD, Box 567, Department 2, Santa Barbara, CA 93102.

✓ Contact the Bureau of Consular Affairs, State Department, Washington, DC 20520, (202) 647-1488 to identify the embassy or consulate closest to where your relative will reside. The Bureau can also give you information on air ambulance services and health insurance companies providing international coverage.

✓ Ask your relative to send you a list of persons you can communicate with in case of emergency.

GLOSSARY OF TERMS

and

APPENDICES

....

GLOSSARY OF TERMS

Accessory Apartment. A private apartment within the structure of a single-family home.

Adult Day Care. Facilities providing a supportive and therapeutic environment during the daytime for older persons with physical or mental impairments.

Advocacy. Activities geared at changes or reforms in systems, policies, or programs.

Aging Network. A system of federal, state, regional, and local agencies providing services for the elderly.

Assessment. A process to determine the physical, emotional, financial, and psychological needs of the older person.

Assisted Living Facilities. Sometimes referred to as *board and care homes*, these houses provide a room, meals, medication supervision, assistance with personal care, and 24-hour supervision.

Care Log. A journal to help caregivers keep track of important information concerning the older person. Care Logs may be purchased from the publisher (see order form at back of book).

Care Management. A process of assessing an older person's needs, identifying services to meet those needs, and monitoring the system of care put in place.

Caregiver Programs. Support activities offered by organizations to assist persons who care for elderly individuals.

Caregiving. Provision of support with tasks related to maintaining the physical and mental well-being of persons who need assistance.

Community Residential Facilities. Also known as *board and care homes, foster homes,* and *assisted living facilities,* this housing offers shared common space, private sleeping quarters, assistance with personal care, meals, medications management, and laundry services.

Congregate Living Facilities. Senior housing that offers independent living, central dining, and a host of recreational and health programs.

Consular Officer. Located at many service posts in foreign cities, these persons are responsible for aiding Americans traveling or living abroad.

Durable Power of Attorney. A power of attorney that remains in effect if the older person becomes incapacitated.

Durable Power of Attorney for Health Care. A power of attorney that gives another person the authority to make health care decisions.

Echo House. A small, temporary house built in the back or on the side of a main home.

Foreign Nationals. Citizens of countries other than the U.S.

Guardianship. A legal process whereby the courts give a person authority to manage another person's personal and/or financial affairs because that person is no longer able to do so.

Home Health Care. A variety of health services that are brought into the home, including medical services and personal care services like bathing and grooming.

Homemakers. Homemaker aides assist with light housework, laundry, ironing, and cooking.

Informal Network. Families, friends, and neighbors who provide unpaid assistance to older persons.

Information and Referral. A service that provides information about aging issues and refers inquirers to programs that meet their needs.

Living Will. A legal document that allows a person to specify the withholding of life support treatments.

Long-Term Care Insurance. An insurance that provides financing for nursing home care and other long-term care services. These policies are useful to older persons who have substantial assets to protect.

Medicaid. A federal/state health insurance program for low income elderly, and blind or disabled persons of any age. Eligibility guidelines vary from state to state.

Medicare. A federal health insurance program for older Americans administered by the Social Security Administration. Part A covers hospital care and Part B covers doctor fees.

Medigap Policies. Medicare Supplemental Insurance, or "Medigap," is private insurance that pays the portion of medical bills not paid for by Medicare. Medigap policies only cover charges approved by Medicare as medically necessary.

Nursing Homes. Institutions offering 24-hour nursing services or supervision, meals, laundry, personal care, recreation, nursing services, administration of medications, and therapies.

Nutrition Sites. Noontime meals offered in a central location such as a senior center, church or synagogue, community center, or housing project.

Older Americans Act. The federal legislation that established a system of services for the elderly.

Ombudsman. A person who investigates consumer complaints in community resident facilities and nursing homes.

Personal Emergency Response Systems (PERS). These systems allow an older person to transmit a signal of distress to emergency telephone numbers. PERS can be a device worn around the neck or a device placed in the bathroom or bedroom.

Power of Attorney. An instrument that gives someone else the authority to act on behalf of another person. A power of attorney becomes invalid when either party becomes incapacitated.

Qualified Medicare Beneficiary Program. A state program administered by state and local departments of social services that pays Medicare premiums, deductibles, and coinsurance for persons with limited income and resources.

Representative Payee. A program that allows a person to receive government benefit payments on behalf of another person who is not capable of managing the payment.

Respite. A period of temporary relief of caregiving duties.

Senior Centers. Places where seniors go to participate in health, recreational, and educational programs.

Springing Power of Attorney. A power of attorney that goes into effect only when a person becomes incapacitated.

Support Groups. Informal groups of caregivers who meet to provide emotional support to one another and to participate in educational activities.

Trust. A document that allows an older person to transfer assets to a legal entity called a trust to benefit another person.

Will. A legal instrument whereby a person identifies who will receive his assets after his death.

National Resource Organizations

Alzheimer's Association
919 North Michigan Avenue
Suite 1000
Chicago, IL 60611
(312) 853-3060; (800) 272-3900
(patients & families only)
The Alzheimer's Association assists
family members of Alzheimer's Disease patients by offering numerous
resource materials.

**American Association of Homes
for the Aging (AAHA)**
901 E Street, NW, Suite 500
Washington, DC 20004
(202) 783-2242
A national membership organization of non-profit elderly housing
organizations. AAHA offers a series
of brochures on housing options for
the elderly for $1.00.

**American Association of Retired
Persons (AARP)**
601 E Street, NW
Washington, DC 20049
(202) 434-2277
AARP is a nonprofit membership
organization providing a number of
free publications for caregivers.

**American Diabetes Association
(ADA)**
National Center
1660 Duke Street
Alexandria, VA 22314
(703) 549-1500; (800) 232-3472

ADA is a voluntary health organization concerned with diabetes. The
association offers brochures on
various topics related diabetes.

**American Health Care Association
(AHCA)**
1201 L Street, NW
Washington, DC 20005
(202) 842-4444
(800) 321-0343 (publications only)
AHCA is an association for nursing
homes. The organization distributes
free brochures on selecting and
paying for nursing homes.

**American Parkinson Disease
Association (APDA)**
60 Bay Street, Suite 401
Staten Island, NY 10301
(718) 981-8001; (800) 223-2732
APDA is an association that
provides information and referral,
public education, and counseling on
Parkinson's disease. The organization offers information and referral
services for caregivers.

Catholic Charities USA
1731 King Street, #200
Alexandria, VA 22314
(703) 549-1390
Catholic Charities USA is a nationwide network that offers respite,
chore services, caregiver retreats,
adult day care and meals on wheels.

Center on Rural Elderly
Univ. of Missouri — Kansas City
5245 Rockhill Road
Kansas City, MO 64110
(816) 235-2180
The Center provides information and referral and self help materials to family caregivers.

Foundation for Hospice and Homecare
519 C Street, NE
Washington, DC 20002
(202) 547-6586
The Foundation offers a free publication on how to choose hospice and homecare agencies. To receive the brochure, send a stamped, self-addressed business envelope.

Health Insurance Association of America (HIAA)
1025 Connecticut Avenue, NW
Suite 1200
Washington, DC 20036
(202) 223-7780
HIAA is a membership organization for insurance companies. The association offers free publications on how to evaluate long term care and Medigap insurance policies.

Medic Alert Foundation International
2323 Colorado Avenue
Turlock, CA 95380
(209) 669-2402; (800) 344-3226
The Foundation offers personal emergency response systems and medical alert bracelets and neck chains.

National Academy of Elder Law Attorneys
655 N. Alvernon Way, Suite 108
Tucson, AZ 84711
(602) 881-4005
The Academy is membership organization for elder law attorneys. It offers a free brochure on how to choose an elder law attorney.

National Association of Private Geriatric Care Managers
655 N. Alvernon Way, Suite 108
Tucson, AZ 86711
(602) 881-8008
NAPGCM is an association of private practitioners who provide care management services for the elderly.

National Association on Area Agencies on Aging (N4A)
1112 16th Street, NW, Suite 100
Washington, DC 20036
(202) 296-8130; (800) 677-1116
(Eldercare Locator Service)
N4A is a membership organization for the 670 Area Agencies on Aging across the country. It offers the Eldercare Locator Service, a nationwide service to help caregivers find community services for the elderly.

National Council on the Aging
409 Third Street, SW
Washington, DC 20024
(202) 479-1200
NCOA is a national , nonprofit membership organization. It offers a number of useful publications for caregivers.

National Institute on Aging (NIA)
9000 Rockville Pike
Bethesda, MD 20892
(301) 496-4000
The NIA, part of the National Institutes on Health, is a federal government's principal agency that distributes free resource materials including a series of fact sheets on aging, called *Age Pages*.

National Stroke Association
300 East Hampden Avenue,
Suite 240
Englewood, CO 80110
(303) 762-9922; (800) 787-6537
The National Stroke Association publishes a number of brochures to help family members cope with stroke patients.

The Simon Foundation
P.O. Box 815
Wilmette, IL 60091
(708) 864-3913; (800) 237-4666
(patient information)
The Simon Foundation provides public education on incontinence.

United Parkinson Foundation
360 West Superior Street
Chicago, IL 60610
(312) 664-2344
The United Parkinson Foundation offers educational symposia for Parkinson patients and their families.

Vision Foundation, Inc.
818 Mt. Auburn Street
Watertown, MA 02172
(617) 926-4232; (800) 852-3029 (Massachusetts only)
The Foundation provides self-help services to individuals and their families coping with vision impairments.

Visiting Nurse Associations of America (VNAA)
3801 East Florida Avenue
Suite 206
Denver, CO 80210
(303) 753-0218; (800) 426-2547 (referral line)
VNAA offers a toll-free number for family members and professionals to locate a Visiting Nurses Association in their area.

Caregiver Organizations

Alzheimer's Family Relief Program
American Health Assistance
Foundation
15825 Shady Grove Road
Suite 140
Rockville, MD 20850
(800) 437-2423
The Foundation provides grants of up to $500 for caregivers caring for Alzheimer's patients with less than $10,000 in cash assets. Grants can be used for respite care, medications, supplies or adult day care.

Caregivers Program
A. H. Wilder Foundation
919 Lafond Avenue
St. Paul, MN 55104
(612) 642-2055
The Foundation distributes practical information for caregivers on a variety of topics including stress management, coping with emotions, setting realistic expectations and self care.

Caregivers Resource Center
Eastern Connecticut Area Agency on Aging
401 W. Thames Street
Norwich, CT 06360
(203) 887-3561
The center is a library of caregiver resources including films, books, pamphlets and lists of available services. The center also offers caregiver seminars.

Children of Aging Parents (CAPS)
Woodbourne Office Campus
1609 Woodbourne Road
Suite 302A
Levittown, PA 19057
(215) 945-6900
CAPS is a nonprofit membership organization for caregivers. The organization offers information and referral services and publishes a newsletter.

Duke Family Support Program
Box 3600
Duke Medical Center
Durham, NC 27710
(919) 684-2328
(800) 672-4213 (North Carolina residents only)
The Duke Family Support Program is an information resource for families caring for persons with memory loss.

Family Caregiver Support Program
Pennsylvania Department on Aging
231 State Street
Harrisburg, PA 17101
(717) 772-2934
This state-wide program offers financial reimbursement of up to $200 per month to pay for respite care expenses or other support services for caregivers who share housing with the care receiver.

Family Survival Project
425 Bush Street, Suite 500
San Francisco, CA 94108
(415) 434-3388
(800) 445-8106 (California only)
Family Survival Project offers state-wide information and referral, consultation, education, respite care and support groups for family caregivers.

National Federation on Interfaith Volunteer Caregivers
105 Mary's Avenue
P.O. Box 1939
Kingston, NY 12401
(914) 331-1358
The Federation helps in starting local interfaith projects providing direct services to family caregivers.

New York State Office for the Aging
Agency Building 2, Empire State Plaza
Albany, NY 12223
(800) 342-9871; (518) 474-5731
New York state sponsors a number of caregiver resource centers throughout the state. These centers offer resource materials, educational activities and counseling for family caregivers.

INDEX

insurance *100*
insurance documents *53*
insurance policies *49*
international caregiving *99-108*
international relocation *105-107*
irrevocable trust *64*

joint ownership *64*

legal documents *49, 50*
legal options *63-64*
legal planning *60*
legal services *61*
living will *63*
locating missing records *54-55*
long distance calls *18*
long-term care *64*
long-term care insurance *66*

Meals-on-Wheels *42, 44*
Medicaid *43, 64, 65, 68*
medical alert bracelet *100*
Medicare *43, 65, 66*
Medicare Supplemental
   Insurance *66, 68*
medigap *66*
military families *103*
monitoring system *80-81*
monitoring system,
   setting up *74-76*
moving abroad *100-101*

National Association of Area
   Agencies on Aging *37*
nonemergency situations *28-29*

nursing homes *95, 97*
nutrition sites *39*

Older Americans Act *36, 42*
ombudsman *95*

Personal Emergency Response
   Systems (PERS) *41*
power of attorney *63*
private care manager *42*

Qualified Medicare Beneficiary
   Program *65*

refusing assistance *81-83*
relocation *87-97*
representative payee *65*
retirement communities *94*
revocable trust *64*

safe deposit box *56*
senior centers *40*
senior housing *90-95, 97*
springing power of attorney *63*
State Units on Aging (SUAs) *37*
supplemental security income *65*
supportive community housing
   93-94

telephone reassurance *41*
telephone savings *17-18*
train travel *31*
travel tips *25-33*
trust *64*

unreliable help *83-85*
updating records *55*

will *63, 100*

ABOUT THE AUTHOR

Angela Heath holds a master's degree in Gerontological Studies from Miami University. She is a nationally recognized expert on caregiving issues, having worked extensively in the areas of research, public relations, program development and evaluation, and community assessment. Ms. Heath's professional accomplishments include establishing AARP's caregiving program, developing and coordinating national awareness campaigns and materials, designing a national survey on Alzheimer's disease resources, and training hundreds of community groups and organizations on caregiving issues and skills. Angela is the author of numerous books and articles including the first booklet on long distance caregiving (*Miles Away and Still Caring*, AARP, 1986), the first booklet series on corporate elder care (*Caregivers In the Workplace*, AARP, 1987), and the recently completed *Caring for Older Adults* (ABC Clio, 1992). She currently owns a consulting firm in Washington, DC which facilitates diversity and management training, develops resources on aging issues and conducts focus group research. She has lectured extensively in both the United States and Canada.

ADVISORY PANEL MEMBERS

The following individuals reviewed working drafts of this book to assure currency, accuracy and appropriateness for the general reading public.

. . . .

Lynn R. Friss, MSW, is the Manager of Research and Information Programs at the Family Survival Project in San Francisco. She also serves as the Statewide Resources Consultant to the California Department of Mental Health in the Coordination of a statewide system of Caregiver Resource Centers. She is active in aging and family issues and is a past officer of the American Society on Aging. Friss earned a master's degree in social work with a specialization in gerontology from the University of California, Berkeley.

Lorraine Lidoff is Vice President for Programs at The National Council on the Aging, Inc. Programs under her aegis include health promotion, intergenerational projects, adult education, and community service development. She initiated NCOA's work on behalf of family caregivers in the early 1980s and has authored *Caregiver Support Groups in America*, *Respite Resource Guide, Family HomeCaring Guides*, and other materials to help families caring for their older relatives.

Joan Kuriansky is the Executive Director of the Older Women's League (OWL). As Director of OWL, Ms. Kuriansky promotes changes in public policy on federal and state levels. She speaks before Congress, to the press, and lectures extensively on issues facing midlife and older women. She received her law degree from the University of Virginia and holds a master's degree in Urban Affairs. Ms. Kuriansky was named "A Woman of Vision" by the MS. Foundation and was presented one of six 1992 Gloria Steinmen awards.

Evelyn C. Aker is a research assistant in the Survey Design and Analysis Department of AARP. She is also the caregiver for her 94-year-old mother. Evelyn is keenly interested in the topic of long distance caregiving as she will be retiring from AARP in 1993 and moving to another state.

Robyn I. Stone, Dr.P.H., is a Senior Policy Analyst at Project HOPE's Center for Health Affairs, located outside of Washington, DC. She is a nationally-recognized expert on long-term care policy, and has published and lectured widley on issues related to family caregiving to the elderly and disabled.

Linda Jackson is a project director at the National Caucus and Center on Black Aged, Inc. She is responsible for developing national and community-based training programs to benefit older adults and their care providers.

Terry Freeman, M.S.S., is Director of the Employee Assistance Program at The Travelers. In that role she has implemented policies and programs to support employee caregivers, including the facilitation of a caregiver support group that has met continuously since 1986.

Barbara R. Greenberg, MSW, is President of The Philanthropic Group, a New York City consulting and management company that assists individuals, foundations and corporations with their charitable contributions to nonprofit organizations. Greenberg has 20 years experience in the private, nonprofit, and public sectors. Prior to founding The Philanthropic Group, she was Executive Director of the Florence V. Burden Foundation. As an officer of The Travelers Companies she directed the company's Older Americans Program and developed award-winning eldercare and retiree programs that won the corporation national recognition.

PHOTOGRAPHS

All the photographs in this book were taken by Ron Thornton, a Denver-based freelance photographer. Mr. Thornton may be reached by contacting the publisher at (303) 980-0580.

ORDER FORM

American Source Books
PO Box 280353
Lakewood, CO 80228
Phone orders: (303) 980-0580

Please send ____ copies of *Long Distance Caregiving* to:

Name _____

Address _____

City/State/Zip _____

☐ *CHECK ENCLOSED (payable to American Source Books)*
($9.95 per copy plus $2.00 postage for the first book and 50¢
for each additional book)

☐ *CREDIT CARD PURCHASE*
Card Number _____
Expiration Date _____
Signature X _____

☐ I do not wish to order now but please put me on your
mailing list so I can receive information on other books in
The Working Caregiver Series.

. . . .

BULK ORDERS

This book is available at quantity discounts to organizations
and businesses interested in using it for educational or promotional purposes. For further information please contact
American Source Books at (303) 980-0580.

CARE LOG
ORDER FORM

ABOUT THE CARE LOG

. . . .

The **Care Log** is the companion volume to *Long Distance Caregiving*. It is an easy-to-use, timesaving organizer that contains all the forms and exercises you will need in developing an efficient and effective plan of care for your older relative. Packaged in a customized three-ring binder, the **Care Log** is broken down into the seven sections discussed in *Long Distance Caregiving*. Contained in the kit are: assessment work sheets • support network lists • community resources • medications sheet • topics for telephone conversations • family meeting summaries • schedule of tasks to complete • travel organizers, and more.

Please send _____ copies of the *Care Log* to:

Name _____

Address _____

City/State/Zip _____

☐ *CHECK ENCLOSED (payable to American Source Books)*
   ($14.95 per copy plus $3.00 postage for the first kit and $1.50 for each additional kit)

☐ *CREDIT CARD PURCHASE*
   Card Number _____
   Expiration Date _____
   Signature X _____

Send completed order form, and check or credit card information to:

American Source Books / PO Box 280353 / Lakewood, CO 80228
Phone orders: (303) 980-0580

—QUANTITY DISCOUNTS AVAILABLE. CALL (303) 980-0580—